Shooting Stars are the Flying Fish of the Night

Lynn Michell & Stefan Gregory

LINENPRESS

Published by Linen Press, Edinburgh 2013

1 Newton Farm Cottages

Miller Hill

Dalkeith

Midlothian

EH22 1SA

www.linenpressbooks.co.uk

© 2013 Lynn Michell & Stefan Gregory

The rights of Lynn Michell & Stefan Gregory to be identified as the
authors of this work has been asserted by them in accordance
with the Copyright, Designs and Patents Act 1988.

A CIP catalogue record for this book is available from the British Library.

Original Design: Submarine Design, Edinburgh
Cover Design and Typesetting: Zebedee Design, Edinburgh

Printed and bound by CPI Group (UK) Ltd, Croydon, CR0 4YY

ISBN 978-0-9559618-8-5

PREFACE

STEFAN GREGORY

Stefan Gregory fell in love with boats one day at the age of four while dangling his head over the side of a skiff that floated in so-clear-as-to-disappear water, watching a trout in the weed on the stream's gravelly bed. This was flying. He had failed to achieve flying before, launching himself into the air from the tree at the back of his house when faith promised everything but only gave him a black eye and a broken arm, and the first of many trips to casualty.

The idea of cruising around seas and oceans, and even sleeping aboard, had first taken shape in the bottom of the wardrobe where his father kept his sailing books. One could hole up in there, as snug a mooring as any found since, with the imagination free to voyage. Peter Heaton's 'Cruising' had its few photos in the middle – black-and-white bowsprits pointing over bow waves that foamed over modest boats for modest post-war sailors. With the wardrobe door shut, and reading by torchlight, there was a good chance mother would sail straight past.

The mixing of water with these wardrobe-bound sailing experiences only took place on occasional Saturdays when father would hire a dinghy on the river and we criss-crossed from bullrush to bullrush, hauling sheets and readying-about lee-o'. There was one delirious summer when we towed our own, newly acquired old dinghy down to Falmouth to liberate her on the sea. Later, college was within reach of the reservoir where the dinghies went-about, looking down on the plain.

In between these sporadic messings about in boats, somewhere between getting married and our son's arrival, a honeymoon round Anglesey launched Lynn's sailing career. The first day's Force 8 subsided, so on the second day we edged out from behind the massive jetty, to find barely a whisper of wind and a huge Atlantic swell rolling in after the storm. Evening saw us perilously shooting the bar into the Menai Straits on the rollers at lowering tide. As our wave crashed onto the bar, and we sluiced on through the narrow channel, it was either going to be never-again, or as-often-as-possible, for Lynn and sailing. Perhaps what sealed it was the lights reflected on the water from a flood-lit Caernarfon Castle. Coming into a haven is a special feeling.

The first mate is utterly unflappable – quite scarily so. She says it's absolute trust in her skipper. I think it may be Drama School that did it; nothing can be as frightening as that. But anyway, absolute trust can be scary. Especially when you're wondering whether this time you've really screwed up.

Lynn won't do nautical terminology, like *port* and *starboard*. *Left* and *right* are all very well if you know which way the pair of you are pointing. *Port* and *starboard* belong to the boat, whichever way up she is and whichever way she is going. There was a tragic air crash when a stewardess looking aft told the pilot that the right engine was on fire and he shut down the starboard one. Mental stress calls for absolute simplicity. Despite her obstinacy, it would be a terribly poor arrival in port without my first mate. We haven't shipwrecked each other yet. We're still alive to argue the toss. And what are a few scratches on the hull between good friends?

LYNN MICHELL

Although I have been sailing with Stefan for thirty years, I'm not a real sailor. I'm a sham. I want to admit that right at the beginning. My official role on the boat is First Mate but while that's appropriate for my relationship with the skipper, my sailing skills fall far well short of those listed on the certificate. What I know and love about sailing is peripheral to the understanding of engines and bilges and pumps and electrical circuits and navigation. With shameless sexism, on our boat, I regard those skills as male territory. I have great admiration for Stefan who can do all these things and more. I have always had complete trust in my skipper.

I remember, a few years back, there was a barbeque evening for folk on boats in someone's garden in Rodney Bay in the Caribbean. I don't know how we got to be invited because usually we stay away from the drinking-and-socialising crowd. But there we were, and we met some sympathetic travellers. Then it rained. Hard. I took shelter on a bench under a tree, another woman joined me and we got talking. She too was married to a committed, dedicated, skilled sailor. She had initially gone along for the ride and found herself, thirty years later, like me, still sailing. Maybe we had had a glass too many because soon my new friend was being so dismissive about her ability on a boat that I was doubled up with laughter. I had asked her if she was knowledgeable, like her husband, and she snorted.

'It's that or stay at home for two months,' she said. 'I don't even like sailing. Not the travelling part. I like it once we've stopped and the boat becomes a home.'

But I had to make sure she was not being modest.

'But you can handle the boat?'

'Only if I have to.'

'Do you know what to do when the skipper shouts: "Turn her to windward!"' I asked.

'I haven't a clue where the wind is. Ever. And I've been sailing for thirty years. And I don't know what windward means.'

'What about port and starboard?' I asked because 'left' and 'right' seem fine to me.

More hysterical laughter.

'How do you manage?' I asked. 'With only the two of you as crew?'

'I guess. And get yelled at. He does most of the sailing.'

Of course she was making a joke of her ignorance but I still recognised a lot in what she said. Look around harbours and marinas in any part of the world, and there are very few women skippers. There are many solo men, missing their wives who won't sail because it's too uncomfortable. They congratulate Stef on having a wife along with him. And of the few who do sail, I wonder how many are as skilled and confident as their partners? If you watch boats leaving a marina, who is at the helm? Who is down below, tidying up or preparing a meal?

I accept the sexist roles we adopt when sailing because the responsibility of getting us safely from A to B is Stefan's. I take my instructions from him. He will tell you I am willfully disobedient but that's not true. He is the one who is monitoring the way the boat is sailing, listening and looking out for problems, checking that all is well in every department, and making decisions. He is never off duty. I am better downstairs. I am quite happy staggering around a fast-moving, tilted boat, making her safe and sea-worthy and comfortable below. I am responsible for feeding us and don't mind cooking with my back wedged against a cupboard while I juggle pans of boiling liquid and pull bread from the oven. This is my territory and I feel no resentment. It is very different at home.

Of course I prefer to be on deck, watching the ever-changing sky and sea, and despite my downstairs duties, that's where I spend most of my time. I can do the routine stuff like hoisting sails and pulling the right ropes (sheets) when we go about. I'm pretty good at the helm but I do it by instinct; by how the boat feels as she moves through the water. I adjust course if I feel her pulling or struggling, not because I have checked wind and sails or understand why there is a baggy bit in one corner of the canvas. I do get a thrill from keeping her on a course when the wind is almost a gale and we are racing along. Stefan, on the other hand, is forever looking at the tell-tails and tweaking the sails – in a bit, out a bit, back in a bit – and getting the balance just right. In the lightest of light wind, he will mess about with the sails to add almost nothing to our speed through the water until I beg him to start the engine.

As for navigation . . . I can't read a map in the car without turning it round so that the road and the car face the same way. I can't read charts either.

So while Stefan is tuned in to the boat – awake and asleep – and totally absorbed in the business of sailing her, I am more knocked off and in my own world, sitting with my feet trailing over the stern or propped up at the bows while the boat rises and falls in a firm rhythm through the water. I love the sensation of sailing. I love the sea and the sky. I love the solitude. I love dropping anchor in a lonely cove, stripping off and jumping into soothing water. Swimming has always been my therapy. While Stefan has a quick splash, I will swim to the shore or way out to sea and back. Then, as the sun sets, we drink cold beer (if the fridge is working) and eat a simple meal in the cock pit. When we lie in our bunks, we can hear the water splashing against the sides of the boat and the wind settling down to a whisper or picking up to a roar. The boat swings gently on the anchor, this way and that. The anchor chain sometimes groans and moans. Familiar noises that lull you to sleep. In the morning, we wake to a new landscape that looks quite different in the clear light of morning and, before the wind gets up, the water around our boat is a clear window in which shoals of bright fishes dance in unison. I break the glass by jumping in before breakfast. Then I make coffee in a pan because glass cafétieres are not allowed on board. It tastes better at sea than anywhere on land. We are doing what we love.

PART ONE

Hunting Scarlet

CHAPTER 1

Dreaming of a Van der Stadt

AUTUMN 2003

The search for Scarlet was preceded by years of sleeping with the Van der Stadt catalogue on my bedside table. It was required reading before dropping off to sleep.

Having already built a couple of dinghies from reclaimed wood found in Edinburgh skips, I very much liked the idea of building my own cruising boat, but observed that there wasn't much time left over from earning a living.

Stefan is a master of under-statement as you will discover as you read on.Many academics are brains on legs but there is a lot more to Stefan. He has always been a skillful maker-of-things. Like Superman, he goes into his phone box and emerges ready for some daunting project. So he starts this tale in typically throw-away style, not acknowledging the skill that went into building the boats. The first, built with son Louis, was a perfect turtle-shell of a dinghy with russet polished planks. It was used for several years to take the crew out to our Drascombe which we kept at Cramond. The second project was much more ambitious – a replica of an old Ness yawl designed by Ian Oughtred. Stefan bent ten foot lengths of quarter inch wood, fragile and wobbly to exactly fit the curved shape of the hull, holding them in place with dozens of clamps (a job for a ten-handed man) until the glue set. The boat was made of many reclaimed woods – teak, oak, ash (the tiller handle), iroko, spruce. By this stage in his life, Stefan was known around The Grange as the eccentric professor with the wild white hair who carried home on his shoulders massive pieces of wood discarded in skips or found on the pavement waiting for the 'special uplift' (I love that word for household items too big to fit in a wheelie bin). Built into the boat was the solid teak rail out of the Victorian bar of the Queens Hall, chucked out when the place was refurbished. Stefan used it for the gunnels and tiller. I played no part in this year-long weekend and evening activity except to admire the precision with which father and son worked and to register the love and care that went into the boat's creation.

I liked the Van der Stadt philosophy of self-build, fast, light cruising boats. We knew, after a number of close shaves in our first twenty-seven footer, the necessity of being able to get to windward on a lee shore and to know we could scrape into a harbour entrance in time when the tide was fast running out.

Lynn and I were a few years short of retirement and planning to go long distance cruising as soon as the various dependents went independent – dogs, kids, parents – but since they showed no sign of doing so, we decided to jump the gun and buy a boat anyway to get into practice. Yes, we knew that this was not very sensible in terms of finance. It would be better to save our pennies, but psychologically, the idea of gradually working up to the big round-the-world voyage made more sense than buying a boat the day after retirement and before departure.

We wanted a sailing boat that would sail well, would carry enough stuff to allow us to be fairly independent of shore, and which could be managed by just the two of us. Initially we decided to look for an aluminium boat because they have lots of good things going for them – strength, lightness, low maintenance. From the engineering point of view too, aluminium is definitely what a boat ought to be built from, as Van der Stadt explained. There was just one problem; they were like hen's teeth, which cut down our choice when looking for a bargain, and a bargain was what we were going to have to find.

As we searched the web, we found ourselves returning again and again to a description of a fifty foot Sparkman and Stevens ketch, a one-off, owned by an American and kept in Norway. Too much money but not ridiculously too much and perhaps there could be some negotiation. It just so happened that there were cheap flights to Norway. The only trouble was that it was October and the three-hour days would soon be setting in.

Sitting up late one night in the spring (most nights actually) I saw that the very same boat was now in Scotland. We were definitely meant to see it. I searched for other boats that we could look at at the same time and found, in the very same marina, a steel forty-four footer which looked quite nice. Half a dozen other contacts didn't get back to us, or the boats were in South Africa, or their owners had decided not to sell.

The following weekend saw us heading for Argyle.

THE SPARKMAN AND STEVENS KETCH

It's a sunny early spring day on the north west coast but absolutely freezing out of the sun. The marina guy ferries us out to the aluminium boat on its mooring and drops us off. She looked really stunning on the web and still looks beautiful in reality from a distance, still attractive on deck. But do we really want a ketch? You have to understand that in this size range, all our knowledge is theoretical. Maybe a ketch is just what we need, but all those years of sleeping with the Van der Stadt catalogue, and our practical experience of boats up to thirty-eight feet, suggests that ketches are a bit fussy and, given today's modern sail-handling aids, the division of their rig into smaller sails is not necessary anymore. But maybe when you get to fifty plus (boat length and age), a ketch is just what a husband and wife need? We have no way of knowing. The experts disagree wildly and you can't charter a boat like this to find out. Charter boats are what we call 'plastic fantastics' – all from the same mould – and anyway, chartering is so expensive that by the time we had tried all the possibilities, we would be perfectly certain of what we wanted and perfectly unable to buy it.

This boat is big! Not absolutely out of the question, but BIG.

We slide the hatch back and descend a long way into the saloon. She's pretty, but also pretty tatty. Apparently she was built for a Mr. Watson of IBM fame to his very high specs, but that was a little while ago. The design and layout look nothing like the photos. After so much web surfing, we thought we had become adept at constructing an interior from photos but here the reality is far off what we had imagined. The entire galley requires limbo dancing. Headroom is a big thing; I'm six-four and although this boat has six-six headroom, that's only if you don't need to cook. The rest of the boat is rather worn with lots of white dust coming off the aluminium. A good design generally though not for us, I think, and Lynn agrees, but it's been instructive because we get a feel for a boat of this size.

After being picked up again, we head for the steel 44. Our ferryman/broker doesn't seem too keen himself on the aluminium boat and mentions a couple of others that we might look at.

Oh my goodness, are we really contemplating buying this air-strip of a boat? This is the first time I have stood on the deck of a boat this size. It is about a mile from the steering wheel to the front tip. How am I supposed to get this into a tight parking space in a marina? She is massive. There are big 38 ft boats and small 38 ft boats. Our 38 ft Bavaria is of the small variety with a good part of the length taken up by a big bathing platform at the back. She is a neat, modern, unchallenging rather boring kind of thirty-eight footer with a few steps down to the modest sized cabins. This monster is 48 ft and twice as heavy. From the deck, she feels daunting.

Inside, she is a big mess. Stefan insisted, before we set out on this quest, that I look beyond mess and dirt and bags of sails heaped up on bunks because all that Is mendable, like you don't worry about the colour of the wall paper when buying a house. How about rust? There is a pale patina on the surface of the aluminium like icing sugar. In the corners it's quite thick. I point it out to Stefan and he nods. The galley is built up against the curving side of the boat so that I can't reach the far side of it. We exchange glances and, with relief, I know he has ruled her out.

A bit of a reality check, this. Other sailors have glibly told us that if you can sail a 38 footer, you can sail a 48 footer, but I'm not convinced. Afterwards, alone, we talk and worry about her size and the rust. Despite her pedigree, we cross the Sparkman and Stevens off our list.

THE STEEL 44

The steel boat is out of the water, a lovely double chined hull with a shiny paint job. Deep fin keel. Steely but speedy. But the owner has a look of desperation. He bought the boat for a long-planned round-world trip but his hopes were dashed when his wife became seriously ill. He has to sell up. We climb the ladder, and into the stern-cockpit where we see that she is gracefully rusting away. Steel boats rust from the inside out. OK, much of the rust is superficial, but still depressing, and her size confirms our belief that we want slightly more boat than this. A pity, because she has a good design with the engine, unusually, slotted under the saloon table. And we feel sorry for the sad skipper and would love to help him by buying his boat.

Poor skipper. His face speaks of sorrow. I find it hard to concentrate as he shows us round his beloved boat. A boat he doesn't want to sell. It is a total tip inside with stuff everywhere. Lone men seem able to live in boats that resemble garages that haven't been tidied for twenty years – bits of boat lying next to coffee cups and packets of biscuits and spare anchors. There is no demarcation between maintenance and living. I try to look past all that, as instructed. But my sympathy for the skipper doesn't hide the rust. Lots of rust. We can't even consider it.

THE OYSTER
We look quickly at a wooden 48 foot Oyster as we happen to be here. Oysters are up towards the Rolls Royce end of the continuum. In fiberglass she would be totally out of reach, and as it is she is still too dear. She is a lovely modern work of wood and glue, and the owner happens to be on board. He is just completing a major refit. Some interesting conversation ensues. He has replaced the whole transom, and I ask him why. A long story about late night reversing.

Wood is good for the soul.

I'm distracted and intrigued by the details below deck that make this boat a beautiful home. It looks clean and organised; comfortable and welcoming. There are pretty cushions and good lighting and a net over the galley dangling dozens of oranges. I tune out of the technical conversation between Stefan and the skipper because we aren't about to buy this boat. Yes, the wood is gorgeous.

THE RIVAL 48
Next we take a quick look at a Rival 48 which is priced at twice our absolute maximum budget. The owner has reached 70 and is downsizing and we

are told that the price is completely unrealistic and that it might go for not much more than half. As if the task of choosing a boat weren't difficult enough already, we now discover that a boat's listed price is not necessarily much indication of its actual price. This boat looks straight out of the showroom. Rivals have a tremendous reputation for long-distance cruising, but this one has a centre-cockpit which, from experience, we don't like. Our first ever boat share had one but we've been sailing stern-cockpits ever since and are not likely to change back. Lynn says centre cockpits make her feel a bit claustrophobic. She likes to trail her legs out of the back. So – apart from the centre cockpit and the list price – this would do very nicely. An interesting boat all told and she turns out to be something of a benchmark for our later deliberations.

THE VAN DER STADT 48

That's it for the Argyll coast. There is one more we want to look at in the Clyde before going home but we know that this one is very special, and we are viewing her just to satisfy our curiosity. This is a Van der Stadt 48. The price is even more seriously over budget and it isn't going to go for a third, but after all those years of sleeping next to that catalogue, we can't turn down this rare chance. We won't waste much of their time.

This is the alpha-boat in a very large marina. She is only five years old and immaculately fitted out. Standing on deck takes the breath away, even more so when you look up the near eighty feet of mast. Down below is equally boat-show beautiful, but much to my surprise, not for us. Van der Stadts are often individually tailored. On this particular boat, the two aft cabins in the quarters under the cockpit have been squeezed so much that I'm not even sure I could contort myself into one of them. It's because, like many modern boats, the sleeping quarters have been squeezed at the expense of a huge saloon. The master cabin forwards is beautiful, and the navigation station quite out of this world. But the internal layout is for throwing parties in marinas, not sailing around the world. We console ourselves that this beautiful boat is not for us. Sour grapes?

Wow! This is an up-market apartment that happens to be on water. There are leather sofas and leather swivel chairs; TV and sound system. The kitchen is positively elegant with marble counter tops and a floor-standing, front opening fridge instead of the usual sort which you jump and dive head-first into. There's a wine cooler. I want to play on the shiny high-tech gadgets in the Nav Station. The bedroom is like a room in a luxury hotel though how do you stay tucked under the sheets of a central bed when the wind blows? The only place to sleep securely is in one of the two stern cabins, but they are for the minions. Squashed and underground. This boat has 'entertainment' written all over it but we don't entertain. We sail and drop anchor in the most isolated bay we can find. Stefan has insisted I don't stare at the decor but this boat is all decor. I must remember to ask him what she would be like to sail.

So that was boat hunting in Scotland. After a great deal more web browsing, we turned our attention southward where the list of boats for sale is much longer. Then, when we started looking even further afield, we realised that boats anywhere in Britain are really expensive compared to other countries. Holland seemed cheaper, and the US cheaper still.

But there was to be one more diversion that summer in the hunt for the boat.

Chapter 2

Moby Dick

SUMMER 2004

This boat hunting opportunity arose partly from a conference I had been invited to attend in Chicago. Still looking for an aluminium boat, we had found a beautiful Sparkman and Stevens, 51 footer, another one-off, in Maine. The web photos promised that she was sleek, black, and altogether alluring.

I phoned up the broker. No, he didn't know exactly what the headroom was but he was six-two and had ample room, and he would get the owner to measure. Various cyber skills distributed around the family led to a plan of the interior, enlarged from the web, that suggested the headroom was 6' 5" maximum. Too close to rely on. I could stop off in Boston on the way back from Chicago and do a detour to Maine. Of course, they had a queue of people waiting to see the boat.

By the time I left, things had shifted around a bit in my favour. The owner and family would be on the boat in Nantucket and were happy to take me for a day's sailing and drop me off somewhere on the mainland of Cape Cod in the evening. A burst on the web had a car booked and ferry schedules sorted. Off I went to Chicago ever-so focused on conference matters.

*

In Boston airport late afternoon, I pick up a hire car and drive out to Hyannisport, only realising, as the traffic thickens, that it is a bank holiday. The drive is not too bad, but finding a room is absolutely impossible so I spend an uncomfortable night in the car before boarding, on foot, the 5 a.m. passenger ferry to Nantucket.

Moby Dick is one of my favourite novels; has been ever since I spent an Easter week with some college friends on the Norfolk Broads with the Home Service serialising Melville's classic just after pub closing time each evening. Nantucket was the homeport of Captain Ahab's ship the Pequod.

My first Nantucket delight is breakfast in the Even Keel; diners are one of my favourite American institutions. Then off to the marina office, and a jump into the moorings launch to ride out to see the boat. I am cordially greeted by the owner, his wife, daughter and her college friend. My host offers an immediate tour of inspection around the deck and I like what I see. She lives up to her web impression, and more.

There are two companion ways: the usual one at the back from the cockpit into the boat, but instead of going down into the saloon, it enters the rear owner's cabin. Then there's a passageway forward to the saloon, though the galley. The bottom of the second companionway comes down from the deck forward of the spray hood (or dodger as they say in these parts). There's a strong camber to the deck which means that the coach house blends into the boat – both hall marks of a Sparkman and Stevens design.

This boat is unusual in that there are two cabins forward of the saloon, one each side of the midline, with a sliding partition between them, with a head forward of the two. Since they can open onto the saloon, this creates a huge amount of space, but space that can be divided up at sea.

But there's a slight problem: standing up. In the tallest part of the saloon, underneath the forward companionway, the ceiling is an inch into my head. My heart sinks. I explain that the broker was adamant about there being more headroom. The owner is as annoyed with the broker as I am. All that way for nothing – except a sail.

We're heading for the diesel pier and then out into Nantucket sound. The day is beautifully clear and warm though there isn't as much wind as there might be for a really good sail. The daughter is curled up in her sleeping bag with a book in the mini cockpit at the top of the forward companion way, shielded by the smaller of the two spray hoods. She explains that this is always the most sought-after roost on the boat.

I take the helm. The wind is blowing less than 10 knots, but with such a tall rig the boat sails well. The speed builds up to 5 knots with enough momentum to keep it moving regardless. The wheel is large and sensitive. Unlike most wheels, it's got 'feel' almost like a tiller. The boat is happy close hauled at not more than 35 – 40 degrees off the true wind. This is a thoroughbred. This is a whole lot more boat than I've ever sailed.

The owner is very helpful considering the ridiculous circumstances. He understands that at least I can learn something about this sort of boat, even if I'm not prepared to have a couple of vertebrae surgically removed so that I can buy and sail this particular one. I have a good snoop around and can't find a single thing wrong except the headroom. Oh, and it transpires that the draught is *two feet* greater than in the advertisement at a massive ten feet. Ten feet is far too deep for cruising in many parts of the world. She seems to suffer problems in the vertical dimension, too far down, not far enough up. But this is the kind of boat we're looking for. They do exist!

They drop me off in Martha's Vineyard for a ferry back to Hyannisport. Another night in the car, and then a beautiful day driving slowly back along the coast, pottering around some of the harbours, on up to Boston, and the flight home.

The slack day gives me time to enjoy the experience and to think that if there are such things as near misses, then somewhere there must be a hit.

CHAPTER 3

⚓

As the days shorten

WINTER 2004

Some months later I'm musing about boats, looking out on cold, grey, damp Edinburgh gardens. So, if we buy one in the US, what do we do then? We have to pay VAT on it to bring it back home, quite apart from a small matter of 3000 miles of pond. Silly idea! We should go back to looking at European boats.

Edinburgh winters are horrible, and the summer has barely been distinguishable this year. The boat share in the Med, which became a family fixture for about a decade, began because Lynn could not cope with Scottish 'summer' sailing. A two week charter trip up the north west coast and islands, caught in the thrall of a Hebridean stationary depression, finally put paid to that. Three out of four of us arrived back with the onset of flu and Lynn said, 'Never again!' However, the Med is not far enough south for escaping the Edinburgh winters. So suppose we kept the boat in the Caribbean instead? We could take our holidays at Christmas? Why worry about bringing the boat back? Who wants it back? Just keep it out there!

Nah! The Caribbean's for the wealthy. It's impossibly expensive to keep a boat there, and you have to get out in hurricane season. But a holiday in the Caribbean this Christmas? Now that sounds like an attractive proposition and of course we would have to go and see what it was like out there if we were thinking . . . wouldn't we? And we could look at boats while we were there, just for homework naturally. We'd have to rent a room because chartering in the Caribbean would be way over budget but we can imagine just how pleasant it would be sailing, should one happen to have a boat, instead of being stranded ashore. The browser turns up something called Serendipity House with rooms to rent on Tortola in the British Virgin Islands, and then it finds a 53' cutter called *Quietly*. Love the name! Mistress Quietly. So the next quest begins.

Quietly, as far as can be gleaned from the information on the website is a stately lady with a plastic bottom. Perhaps we have to give up the aluminium idea; it just cuts down the possibilities too much. *Quietly* is a reasonable price too, something we could manage, at least if the broker is anything like accurate about what the owner would settle for. A lot more searching and we find several more interesting boats for sale in the Caribbean. Tortola seems to be a good base, and there are reasonable island hopping flights and ferries so we could see the other boats in Antigua and the US Virgin Islands. An essential, fact-finding holiday, in fact.

*

Serendipity House is wonderful. It's on the undeveloped north side of the island, about half a mile from the sea, and was built as a guest house to the main house. There is no air conditioning, but everything we need in one Caribbean pink and purple room. The beach is a twenty minute walk down the hill and just out of this world – warm sea and mountainous rollers pounding the beach. And scary-sized pigs on the shore! Immediately after arriving we rush down to swim in a gentle drizzle. That night we find that we pallid ones managed to get sunburnt in the rain. What happens in full sun?

This is serendipity indeed. We've landed ourselves a candy-coloured bedroom plus kitchen with a balcony where we practise our newly learned yoga – if we can stop gawping at the view of tropical forest and rainbows. Rain and sun. Heat and damp. Utter peace. I sometimes forget we are here to eye up boats.

MISTRESS QUIETLY

For a couple of days we play in the surf to recuperate, and then we take the ferry to Anagorda where *Mistress Quietly* is berthed. She's out of the water with her keel sunk in a hurricane pit so that her water line is at ground level which makes her look like a large cow lying down grazing in a field of grass surrounded by the rest of the herd. She looks great. Not as sleek as your Sparkman and Stevens but elegant nevertheless. Immediately, we are up the ladder, undoing the hatch, and descending into the interior. A bit of a mess with her gear piled everywhere. A good layout, and bags of space. Looking at boats you get used to a muddle and you have to see through it. But *Mistress Quietly's* muddle puts me on my guard – not quite healthy muddle perhaps.

I take up the first few floorboards. There's always a horrendous maze of wiring, pipes, god-knows-what. They call them 'systems' in the magazines. *Quietly* is serene in her exterior but anything but peaceful in her bilges. She's also really big. Her layout is excellent, designed for sailing rather than parties, but I can see that Lynn is ruling her out as a serious proposition. I'm a bit more reluctant to come to a decision, but those bilges, full of more wires than the European telephone system, are not exactly encouraging. We talk further to the broker about exactly what price the owner would take, but it's not low enough to fix what needs fixing, even though what needs fixing is apparently fairly superficial.

Why is my husband spending hours and hours creeping over and around and under this boat, lifting hatches and poking at the engine and spuddling in the bilges? She is a mighty beached whale wallowing in grass instead of sand and at first sight I don't like her one bit. She is formidable. He can't be serious? I'm taking in the big picture while he is mucking about with details like the complexity and muddle of the wiring. The electricity cables are trailing in the bilges! This is one impossible and unwanted project. She is a train wreck inside and I'm not talking cosmetic repairs. She needs cleaning up and re-building on a scale I'm not prepared to take on. Virtually all the wood – and there is a lot – needs to be sanded down and varnished and in places replaced. Around every port hole the aluminium is badly corroded. They would all need to be replaced. The heads (loos) are small, stinky and revolting. The galley needs a complete re-fit. Too much. Far too much.

As I said earlier, my husband is not a pushover when it comes to arguments. He persuades me that re-building and re-furbishing would not be not impossible if we can get her at the right price. I tell him we will spend more years on maintenance than sailing and may be dead by the time the project is finished. And how do we work on her when she is beached on Virgin Gorda? Fortunately the price isn't right and I breathe a silent sigh of relief.

THE FIRST MASON

Back in Tortola, it's one of those roasting days where the air is too hot to breathe and you daren't move in case you expire. We're in a marina consulting another list of boats, when Lynn sees the Mason. Its air conditioning is running. It's almost icy cool inside and it is love at first sight. Lynn flops down on one of the white settees, recovering.

This boat is very light and airy with none of *Quietly*'s water stains or corroding aluminium port lights. Masons are heavy duty cruising boats, beautifully built to high specs and this one, though twenty-five years old, looks like a five-year old boat. A serious wraparound galley with a bum-strap for dynamic cooking; strong bronze and stainless steel deck fittings; an incredibly compact design. She is appreciably smaller than anything else we have seen and really and truly not big enough. There is a double cabin at the front and at the back a double berth which fills the entire cabin leaving very little storage space except underneath.

The headroom inside is OK, but it is achieved at the expense of a too upright box of a coach roof which takes away deck space. I love the boat but feel it isn't the sort of boat we had set out for. She has oodles of soul, but not enough cabin sole.

This is a heavy long-keeled downwind boat but one in which I would not want to beat to windward. Of course this judgment is as theoretical as the rest of our knowledge in this size range, but 44 is near enough to the 38 that we knew well for me to have a fairly firm belief that Lynn would be quite frustrated. There are those who will tell you that you don't need to beat to windward while cruising, but it seems to happen to us quite regularly. Besides, the adrenalin addict would not get her regular juice. Lynn doesn't see it that way immediately, perhaps seduced by the cool air and the white settee.

It is a midday tropical boiler-house outside – a heavy dripping debilitating heat – when we step down inside this pretty, immaculate boat. It is cool inside. Really cool. This is my first time in an air-conditioned boat and I am enraptured. I lie down on the white settee and enter boat heaven. Once my body reaches a normal temperature, I look around, admiration building to adoration. The stern master cabin is small but the bed is big, built up against the wall, and has storage space underneath. It feels very comfortable, like a real double bed. OK, I'll have to take fewer clothes. No problem. The kitchen is a perfect U-shape of useable, safe space, well equipped with lots of thoughtful detail. I would not be thrown across the boat while moving pans of bubbling pasta and cheese sauce. The saloon's squashy white sofa circles the polished table on one side and the long sofa-for-stretching-out-on faces it. There is a spotless, modern shower-room and another cabin in the foc's'l. This boat is perfect. Not too big. Not too small. Just right. And cool.

Why is Stefan not enthusing over this boat? Why is he so quiet? He listens to my eulogy but I know he is patting the head of a silly child and soon I will be told the nasty truth. He is not even going to consider it. I sigh and grieve over his conclusion but there is no budging him.

THE SECOND MASON

Next day, while checking out marinas for their fees, we happen across another Mason, the same model but a couple of years older, done up as his labour of love by a wealthy and engaging American retiree, and incredibly beautifully built and rebuilt she is. He is only too pleased to show us around his handiwork, even though he is never going to sell her. So we really get the inside story on Masons, and a very good story too, but not quite our story. And, incidentally, the marina fees are expensive, but not totally prohibitive. By staying away from the fashionable marinas it might be possible to get costs down to not much above Croatia or at home. We hear that fixing boats with anything but the most routine of problems could be difficult, slow, and expensive on the smaller islands, but in Tortola, where there is one of the biggest charter fleets anywhere, what couldn't be fixed would stay broken, worldwide.

THE CARDINAL 46

Then there was the one we missed. A Cardinal 46 on Tortola which had tickled our antennae back home on the web, was sold out from under us the week before, and no, we couldn't see her out of interest, and they weren't even going to tell us where she was.

THE HINKLEYS

Our final trip was to the USVI Island of St Johns to see a number of Hinckleys, another traditional American cruising boat, one of the few still being built in the US. Hinkleys are a little like Masons but are centre boarders, lighter and beamier, but also very beautifully put together. They were designed as a result of a history of cruising rather than because a salesman was told to maximise berths. The particular boat we went to see was not definitely for sale. It was the pride and joy of the owner of the marina who had arrived by this very boat back in the 60s and had now accumulated a whole mooring full of Hinckleys and their owners. He was amazingly generous with his time and showed us not just his own boat, which was beautiful but even smaller than the Mason, but also half a million's worth of Hinckley 50+. As with all such mornings spent, we learnt a lot from our kind host.

After that it was back to Tortola and Serendipity, and one last dip in the surf that still pounded the beach.

Our trip had persuaded us that the Caribbean didn't seem quite so completely out of the question as the place to keep our boat. We had often discussed the fact that the economics would change radically once we retired and lived full time aboard, abroad. One of the main costs is marina fees and when we cruise, we mostly avoid marinas. The need to get out of the summer/autumn hurricane season was one of the chief problems but one possibility would be to lower the boat into a hurricane pit, like *Quietly*, and another to take the boat to Grenada, Trinidad, or even the Venezuelan Islands which are further south than the hurricane track.

Quietly had lured us out there, and *Quietly* wasn't quite right, at least without a major price-reduction, but it had been a very enjoyable learning experience.

And so back home to Scotland, the dark, and e-hunting instead of boat ogling. The search continued.

CHAPTER 4

More Cardinals and some white smoke

JANUARY 2005

It's the New Year and we are still at the web browsing.

We toyed with the idea of a *Quietly* clone in San Diego. I would have to brush up on the Panama Canal. *Ocean Passages of the World* assures us that it would be a wonderful trip down Baja, but a bit of a beast from there onwards. Hawaii and back the other way would be more plausible, but isn't this getting out of hand? If we were going to retire straight away, then California would make sense as a purchase place for setting off into the South Seas. But sailing back across the Pacific on annual holidays? Get real!

Some more homework on Cardinals suggests that on Tortola we had had a close encounter with what might be the right boat for us. Cardinals, it turns out, were designed by Alan Warwick, a New Zealand yacht designer, who has designed all sorts of boats from Americas Cup yachts on down. I read somewhere that the Cardinal's hull was made in the old moulds from the Swann 47, a Sparkman and Stevens design. That designer again! I have no idea whether it is true but it sounds like a good pedigree. The Cardinal has a seriously sexy hull anyway – no great bum at the back that doubles as a bathing platform – partly an aesthetic matter, but also about the way a hull sails. The huge wide sterns on modern charter boats allow two quarter cabins to be crammed in, and they go like stink downwind, but when the boat heels on the wind, they create too much weather helm, and

27

generally spoil the helm's feel. The older elegant counter sterns don't offer as much room inside, and they don't make good swimming platforms. They are slower downwind because they tend to 'bury'. But when they heel, the helm stays true.

As well as the usual Sparkman and Steven double companionways, the Cardinal has an almost unique arrangement whereby the navigation table is in the owner's stern cabin, right next to the companionway into the cockpit. Right where it is needed. That appeals to me. The common Sparkman & Steven design for this rear cabin has two single bunks, one each side, whereas other Cardinals, this one included, has a big double bed on one side, and the navigation station on the other. I could get into this. At least, after magnifying the plans and measuring, it looks as if I might get into this.

Denied one Cardinal, the hunt was on for another, and not just because we had missed one. It transpired that only a few had been built. The next Cardinal we found was in Florida and was all set up for cruising. It had been cruised seriously, and seemed to have the stuff on board that we would need, and not too much that we wouldn't. It was a bit too much money, but not too much too much. We contacted the broker. It had gone. They don't seem to hang around, these Cardinals. Every other boat we had seriously considered had been on the market for months. Two Cardinals disappeared just as we found them. On one of the chat rooms on the web I stumbled on some guy sounding off about how this was the only boat for him and he was determined to get one. I didn't join in.

We found two more, one for double our price in Connecticut, and one a bit cheaper than the one we just missed – and in Florida. I started compiling every bit of information I could get, blowing up the plans and measuring the headroom. Six foot seven! I liked what else I saw too. Yes, this was ridiculous. We were just back from the Caribbean, Christmas was just gone and we'd never even seen one of these Cardinals in the flesh. I got in touch with the Florida broker and he told me it had gone – cheap. Apparently there were some problems. It was a trade boat – one bought by a broker in part exchange for another boat. Brokers are keen to explain how many problems there are with a boat once it has been sold. But there was one bit of interesting news; the one in Connecticut has been on the market for ever because the price is crazy. Worth a tilt, he said.

I hate phones. I will go to some lengths to avoid using them. We are the only two remaining people in the UK who don't have a mobile. I particularly hate wheeling and dealing on the phone so it took a while to screw up the courage to phone the broker about a boat advertised at $320,000. It took the previous four Cardinals having sold like hot cakes to get me on the phone rather than doing one more search for some really useful information about the equipment. I went through the routine questions:

How much headroom is there?

How far is it from the floor to the ceiling?

If measured from the ceiling to the floor, what would that be?

Are American inches the same as Imperial inches?

He said he wasn't sure, measured 6' 6" off the plans, and then said he'd have the yard measure it. Yes, he would fax the results in blood by return.

The rest of the call was less fraught. The boat had been tied up at the yacht club for fifteen summers, and in a shed each winter. The owner was beginning to get twitchy about buying another boat in time for spring and beginning to realise that the price he had insisted on was unrealistic. He might just be open to a lower bid if he could sell sooner rather than later. The procedure was to be as follows:

- We agree a price subject to inspection and survey and we pay 10% deposit
- We inspect, and if we don't like, we pull out and get our deposit back.
- If we do like, we survey and if we don't like, we pull out and get our deposit back.
- If we do like, we cough up. Shed fees and launching are included in the price.

It is now January. The temperature in Connecticut is well below freezing. The boat is apparently jig-sawed into a very large shed with twenty other boats, but yes, we can see it if we come out. So can the surveyor. It means we can't sail her before making a decision. The surveyor can't survey the boat properly in a frozen shed, but a percentage of the price is withheld in escrow in case there are problems which emerge when the boat is launched and sea-trialed in the spring. Like she sinks.

So here we are apparently thinking about buying a boat without sailing her or even seeing if she floats.

CHAPTER 5

Spending money is hard work

JANUARY 2005

I make another call to the broker. We go over the procedure. We talk price. It becomes clear that he doesn't have much idea about what the owner will take, but he seems to regard the advertised price as a joke.

What's it worth? It's a whole lot less boat than the Maine too-low-too-deep boat and, apart from being fiberglass, it is a more suitable boat. Twelve tons instead of seventeen. Six foot six instead of ten feet draught. A much smaller engine, just adequate, which is what we like. Slab reefing which is more reliable and sails better instead of in-mast roller reefing. About the same age, but with a whole lot less miles on it. A similar sort of boat with a Sparkman & Stevens type of design making her swift and elegant but also a real cruising boat. Fast and sturdy. Not an easy combination to find. Not a plod, but not an all out racer either. It's about the same in dollars as the Rival 48 was in pounds, and just at the moment, there are nearly two of the former to one of the latter. OK, it is four years older, but lightly used. It's about the same price as where we stopped bargaining on *Quietly*, which was in a much worse state, and not nearly as good a design. Unless there are some hidden elephant traps, this is a bargain. If there are hidden elephant traps, we are the elephants.

Can we do any better? Who knows? Lynn and I decide that we're going to go for this one, subject to the boat being as nice in the flesh as on spec. The broker suggests trying $170,000. We go in at $130K and he goes off to ask the owner who comes back with $165,000. Hmmm! We book flights for the first week in February.

There is a small hiccup. Over the phone it transpires that the photos in the advert are not photos of 'our boat'. I lose my rag. We are supposed to wire $16K to some foreign account for a boat a little like some photos of another boat. On what basis? I start on a philosophy tutorial. What evidence do we have that this boat exists? Is the broker more than an answering machine somewhere in the Gobi desert? I google the broker. There are not one but two brokers with the same name, neither in the Gobi; one in NY and one in CA. Same name, same logo, just different addresses and different boats for sale. So that's all right! That's twice as much existence as a mere one broker. I enquire of the Broker's Association what they know about this firm.

'Well, we're not allowed to tell you anything useful, Sir.'

An unusually frank answer! After some cajoling, the woman on the phone lets slip that the broker has not paid the Brokers Association dues this year. Very encouraging! Nonpayment offers some evidence of existence.

I confront the broker, almost phone-desensitised by this stage, and he explains that the CA firm is an offshoot and that they didn't feel like buying a second expensive logo and that he is allergic to paying fees on time. The philosophy soliloquy starts again. We have no independent evidence of anything so the broker could be the conjuring of an evil genius. I phone the New York Chamber of Commerce and find that at least there is a registered company at said address which has been there for ten years. The broker's bank assures me that any money we pay into that account goes into an escrow account, ie: it doesn't belong to the broker until the boat is ours. More mere phone numbers. Is the New York Chamber of Commerce real? Answer on both sides of the paper! The broker's answering machine assures us that real pictures (more simulacra) of the real boat are to arrive by email soon. The concept of proof-of-purchase takes on a whole new meaning.

OK, enough skepticism. We're off to see if we can kick the rock. We wire the deposit through a currency dealer who saves us more than a thousand pounds on the ten percent deposit which the bank offered. There's reward for twenty year's loyalty for you. The dealer talks an unreal conversation about dollar trends, generally down, with blips. The dollar is dropping towards two to the pound. He thinks it will not be much different, maybe a bit better by March when we have to pay. I said,'When, not if.' Caught myself! So we don't hedge currency. Is this really us?

I am beginning to understand just how much homework goes into buying a boat. Simple tasks, described in a phrase, unpack into baroque procedures with obligatory offerings to the correct gods. She has to be registered. Does this make a difference to our VAT liability? If she is eventually headed for the Caribbean and we don't want to import her into the EU, we don't really want to pay a seventh of her value in VAT for a few months' visit. So what about the British Virgin Islands? There are numerous companies that arrange registration in the BVI for a consideration. When phoned and asked whether this means the boat avoids paying VAT in the EU, they explain that that is a taxation matter and they are not allowed to comment, but (sotto voce), You'll be fine, Mate. I smell a rat, and continue googling until I come across the idea of 'beneficial ownership.' That sounds good; I like the idea that buying a boat as a benefit.

However, 'benefit' here means that although the registration can hide who the beneficial owner is, every time you enter the EU, you have to pretend you are not that owner, which is not a game we're willing to play. It's designed for the professionally crewed Super-yacht, not us, silly! So we opt for a UK Small Ships Register entry and send off the forms and a cheque for £12. We get back the number 116111 which is neat and easy on the memory neurons. Sticky labels with this number are duly ordered. When peeled and stuck on the outside of the boat, we will be legal. I'm getting ahead of myself again.

*

We jump on a plane direct to Newark, hire a car, drive up to Connecticut and check into a motel. Next morning, on early time jet lag, we eat eggy bread doused in maple syrup with a toy train pulling wagons of very late Christmas presents, going round and round on a shelf just below the ceiling of the motel dining room. It is no more surreal than anything else. Then, really nervous because we've kind of set our hearts on this boat though neither of us has admitted it, we set off for the boatyard. We pass by the waterfront and look out to see the Coast Guard icebreaker clearing a channel on the river. We pull up outside the boatyard shed, all piled about by mounds of snow from the blizzard last week, and with a forty foot frozen puddle in front of the main door. This apparently counts as thawing. I am shivering with cold and anxiety and anticipation. This is an awful long way to come on a hunch that this is the right boat.

The broker seems a decent enough sort and we are duly reassured that he isn't just an answering machine. He lets us into the shed and we stoop under all the packed in, stacked up gin palaces until we arrive underneath a wing-keeled, grey, anti-fouled hull. Nothing like meeting the bottom of your future mistress first. The shape is really very fine. Curves taper to an elegant, slightly reverse-counter stern. The anti-fouling looks as if it's been redone since it was in the water.

Up the ladder, we fight through gigantic sheets of polythene, and we're in the cockpit, in the grey light of the mercury lamps way up on the ceiling. A wonderful stern cockpit, long enough for me to lie down in, but small enough to be seaworthy. A huge wheel. A really neat counter stern. Controls and instruments to hand. Acres of teak deck in good shape. We'd as soon not have teak, but if it's there, then it had better be sound. The deck fittings are good and the stanchions and lifelines are rugged. The spinnaker pole is HUGE. In fact everything is distinctly chunky as well as sleek. She weighs just under twice our current 38 foot Bavaria boat share.

I'm holding my icy breath as we limbo dance our way around some mighty ugly gin palaces to arrive in the space underneath our boat. See – I'm writing 'our boat' already. My first response is relief that, from this angle at least, she looks so new, although she is twenty years old. She looks well cared for. Her hull is dark blue and shiny. With freezing hands clinging to its sides, I climb the ladder and stand on deck. A wooden deck that to my untutored eye looks very good indeed. And all the aluminium around all the port holes is shiny not rusty. Polished shiny. I grin at Stef across the miles of teak. I know by now, though, that appearances may be deceptive and that I am no judge of anything other than space and light and appearance. I remember the air-conditioned boat that I bought in the first five seconds of viewing her and know I have to wait for Stef's verdict.

The first thing we see at the bottom of the companionway is the impressive circuit panel in all its glory, mahogany framed with about forty, neatly labeled circuit breakers. Aaargh! There's a spacious double bunk on the left hand side, under the cockpit bench, but with plenty of knee room and without that claustrophobic feeling of being down a hole. It will feel airy lying here, staring up the companionway at the sky and the stars.

I can sit upright in the navigator's table, facing forward. Just.

We go through the tunnel into the galley which is an L shape with the solid gimbaled oven immediately inside the door where you can brace yourself against the engine compartment while you cook. The rest of the galley is well laid out with plenty of counter and cupboards where they're wanted. It is a good width for me. I can brace myself back against the engine compartment and still reach the sink and counter but it will be a bit of a stretch for the real chef.

I can see that the galley is going to be a problem in high seas. It's a spacious L shape with lots of storage, and the gimbled cooker is, like everything else, shiny. I test it out. With my back pressed against a kitchen cupboard, behind which is the compartment for the engine, I am safely positioned to cook on the stove immediately in front. But after that, it's wide open and there is nowhere to brace myself as I move towards the work surfaces and the sink. A tight U shape would be safer. The saloon is very comfortable and welcoming with its somewhat sunken C-settee circling a big table with a hole for the mast. Opposite is a straight settee which pulls out into a generous single berth, long enough for Stef to lie on without his feet and ankles sticking over the edge. And there are plenty of rails to grab on an unsteady voyage at 45 degrees. As for the fo'c'sle cabin, it's love at first sight. It is a high, small padded triangle which I can easily move around on, but it might defeat easy entrances and exits for Stef without a three point turn. Sleep with your head up front and there is room for only one pillow. Mine. Just aft of it is a compact loo with a clean wash basin and a huge gold-framed mirror. I stake it out as my territory. This will be my retreat. Stef can claim the huge captain's bed opposite the nav table right next to the steps leading up on deck. Well, we'll share it.

There is one small feature which makes me wonder about the current owners. On a sort of sideboard at the bottom of the saloon steps is a large and truly ghastly arrangement of plastic flowers.

The boat looks in good shape. Very lightly used. We spend an hour rummaging, admiring mostly, and asking endless questions. A lot of the gear is slightly different from the European equivalents. We look at each other and can immediately tell that we're both sold, which means the broker can probably tell too. It's a good job the price is already agreed.

It's about 10 below in the shed and despite the long johns, it's beginning to get through. Off to the restaurant to thaw out. More endless questions. It turns out that the broker was responsible for importing the boat from Taiwan and for finishing her locally back when he ran a boatyard, so he knows a lot about this particular boat's construction details. He tells us that the owner is a busy man who sails with the family now and again as well as doing some light club racing. Yes, the reading on the hours meter on the engine is genuine; two hundred and fifty hours since new. I work out that if this is true, he has sailed the boat a maximum of eighty times since new. More likely only forty.

We discuss surveying which is all swings and roundabouts. We can independently find a surveyor who may or may not be any good. Or we can accept a recommendation for a good surveyor who may or may not be independent. We decide with some trepidation on the second. We have some experience of random surveyors which isn't encouraging but no experience of dependent ones.

We go back into the freezer of a boat shed, climb back up, and spend another hour or so inspecting and admiring. We admire the mast which is the top one on the rack, forty feet up the shed wall. Of course we can't inspect it because we don't have our climbing gear with us but it is agreed that any faults that can't be found until she is in the water will come under the escrow sum of money withheld until the boat is launched. The jet lag is beginning to set in, and Lynn is a tasteful shade of blue, so we call it a day. We drive in triumph back to the motel to thaw out, and pass out, and spend the next day exploring the estuary in freezing cold, bright sunshine, trying to take in the reality of the situation.

CHAPTER 6

⚓

Long distance dealings

JANUARY 2005

Later that day we drive back to Newark, fly home, and I'm back in the office on Monday morning as if nothing has happened. We commission the surveyor. He surveys and announces everything is hunky-dory with only minor qualifications, and he writes some clauses into the contract about parts of the boat beyond his reach which must be covered by the escrow.

There is a frenzy of activity in our 'spare time.' We nail down the final understandings of what is and isn't included. We have to arrange for payment and insurance. The dollar gyrates wildly and the sterling price falls by about $10K in a fortnight. The company we used for our boat share is pricey, but it is a devil we know. They can cover the boat while it's in the shed, but need a survey to give full cover, which is fine.

Still checking and double-checking, we find another Cardinal 46 on the web, this time in Mallorca, a similar boat but a good deal more expensive, VAT not paid, and with a navigation station in the saloon rather than the Captain's cabin. A weekend in Mallorca anyone?

We decide not. It would be more useful to start some serious planning. If we buy now we would launch in May and:

(a) Sail her back across the Atlantic
(b) Sail her in the US and leave her there over winter
(c) Go uphill against wind and current to the Caribbean.

What is the time window? When does the hurricane season start? What routes are possible? Where can we leave her? Another session with *Ocean Passages of the World* ensues. The mid-Atlantic is a huge spiralling bath tub of water which goes around clockwise, along with the wind. It can be easier to get from New York to Florida with the spiral by going by way of the Canaries than going in a direct line against it. The New York to the Canaries trip is about 2300 nautical miles and is generally an easy route between May and the beginning of the hurricane season which theoretically begins in late June, but the probability of severe storms remains low until mid-July. Once you are farther east than about 50 degrees west, probabilities drop even further and there are no hurricanes at any time east of 30 degrees west at the latitude of the Canaries.

A common route is to sail six hundred miles from the east Coast to Bermuda, then on to the Azores and finally to the Canaries. The goal is to keep far enough north to stay out of the calms in the Azores/Bermuda high, but not so far north that the winds get too strong north of about 45 degrees. So, one heads north from Bermuda to 40 degrees and then east until finally turning for the Azores from the north west. Breaking the trip in Bermuda sounds a sensible plan even if it adds 600 miles. We could find out if we fancied crossing the Atlantic, and head back to the US if we didn't.

These are nature's constraints. What about the human ones? No VAT has been paid on the boat. Google says that the Canaries are VAT free but amazingly the Azores aren't, even though both are Atlantic Island parts of the EU. At about a seventh of the boat's value, VAT is a sizable sum. If we were tax-resident outside the EU for a year, then we could import the boat as goods and chattels, or some such quaint legal phrase, without paying VAT ourselves until we sold it. Perhaps we should keep the boat out of the EU until we retire?

CHAPTER 7

Equipping

JANUARY 2005 ONWARDS

We go through the inventory and establish that the boat lacks some absolutely essential and basic stuff such as a tender and an anchor chain.

She has a rather fancy electric autopilot but no mechanical wind vane self-steering. I don't think long-distance sailing is safe without a wind vane. If the electric goes, you're hand steering 24 hrs a day, not funny with a crew of two or three. There isn't a life raft. I don't think much of life rafts, though my prejudices are theoretical. I just don't fancy my chances once it's a matter of getting into a life raft but if I drowned the family because we didn't have one I'd be pretty low. So we're looking for a life raft. We also need an EPIRB which sends a signal to a satellite which sends a signal to the rescue services showing them where we are – somewhere in the middle of the Ocean – and telling them we would really like to be rescued please. I consider an EPIRB vital and owning one might justify buying a life raft.

Those are the big ticket items. It turns out to be impossible to get any accurate information out of either the broker or owner about what, in reality, is on the boat. At various times we have a Danforth anchor, a Bruce anchor, no anchor but chain, no chain but warp. The same goes for sails. A blade jib appears and disappears. The running backs and inner-forestay likewise (no, we knew there was no American football team on the foredeck but it wasn't so clear whether we'd need them there to weigh anchor).

These running backs are running rigging, important for long distance ocean sailing with a tall rig, but they are, it turns out, absent. Do we need lifejackets and harnesses? Or rather, have we got them? I consider the possibility that they are all rogues, but decide it's more cock up than conspiracy. It still makes hard work of preparations.

Wind vanes are like hen's teeth. No, like Cardinal 46s. They fly off the shelves. Quite a bit of homework involving engineering dimensions of the boat's *derrière* as well as reviews of old salt's attachments to, and for, their vanes, reveals that we either want a Hydrovane or a Monitor. The former is £6K new, the latter about £4K. Even second hand, if you can find one, they go for about 60% of new. That is a lot of money. Already more than it was the week before we paid for the boat. Of course we have already spent more than we should just buying the boat. It'll have to be Ebay.

I spend an awful lot of hours researching the market for wind vane, tender, outboard, life raft, and EPIRB. If I just went down to the shop and bought them new, we would have a bill of more than £10K. Ebay is a whole other world with some strange fauna. Rubber dinghies seem to attract a particular kind of minor fraudster to online money laundering. Wind vanes are different. They just sell in front of your eyes. Then one day I mistype 'wind-vein' and Bob's your uncle, there is one in Texas which has no bids and its auction is finishing. I phone up in a hurry and discuss the ins and outs of a highly complicated piece of engineering which I have never seen. I like the guy. I have an affinity with someone who does the same typos as I do. He is a dealer in boating stuff but seems straight and we come to a deal. Yes, he can ship it to Connecticut insured. Yes, I can pay by PayPal. I type in the passwords, numbers, incantations, and sign away a big dollop of money. Next morning the transaction has bounced. Although it's well within the limit on the card, I have to get PayPal certified. It's a bank holiday and the process involves my bank. I grovel to the guy in Texas. He is very kind but assures me he has others waiting. The folk at PayPal drag it out; we have to test the system by wiring secret small amounts of money known only to them and me to prove that I have access to my bank account. Finally, PayPal is sorted. The guy in Texas has gone to his daughter's graduation and will be away for a week. Maybe he has sold the wind vane to the German he mentioned. Let's hope not! Much later someone tells me there is a dictionary of Ebay typos that one can use to find mislabelled items for sale which have no bids because they have fallen through the category net.

After two fraudsters attempt to sell me nonexistent rubber dinghies on Ebay, I settle for a new one with an outboard from a shop. Ebay is better for life rafts. Maybe the rule is to go for anything that can be spelt with or without a hyphen, with or without a space? If it's the rubber that attracts the perverts to frauding on dinghies, it doesn't seem to have the same effect with life rafts. After watching bidding on a few to get some idea of the price, I find an off-shore, four man one with a double floor (most occupants die of hypothermia, not thirst or lack of food). It needs servicing, but second-hand ones nearly always do. I get up at 3 a.m. to watch the bidding close on the US east coast, and place an absolutely last minute bet – it feels like betting – and dance around the room when I have won, much to the sleepy dogs' bemusement! Now its merely a matter of hoping that PayPal continues to do it's stuff, getting the life raft shipped to a servicer, and thence onto the boat. This all starts amazingly smoothly.

There are no charts on the boat and this causes no end of trouble, partly because we are not sure whether we'll be in the Chesapeake or crossing the Atlantic. There are two chart plotters but getting the specs is as hard as finding out whether we have an anchor. Finding out whether there are to be any charts left on the boat is quite out of the question. Charts are expensive. We don't have any experience of e-charts, but have plenty of experience of being ripped off by software which cuts you off from whatever path of development you wind up wanting to take. A few enquiries and it turns out that sure enough there is a format change between the two generations of chart plotter we have, even though they are made by the same manufacturer, and a further format change since the newer one. There are freely available US Government charts and open source plotting software. It's always an interesting pastime listening to sales people trying to tiptoe around the elephant in the living room and not providing the information you want about whether their software is compatible with the undoctored charts which the tax payer provides. I think the answer is No but I'm still not very sure.

A minimalist approach is a paper plotting chart for the ocean stuff, and local large scale charts of Long Island to Newport, and of the Atlantic Islands. We settle in the end for an Admiralty chart of mid-northern

Atlantic. We would just kiss the ceiling of this chart as we track up a little above 40 degrees. We'll wait until we get to the boat to buy the local stuff. The two chart plotters on the boat have two GPSs, but we buy the cheapest, hand-held, dry battery backup called Gecko. I am later amused as we get into the Azores, one-third of the way across, to realise that, despite the fancy stuff on the boat, we have settled down to navigating by using the Gecko and penciling the readings on to the paper charts. But I'm getting ahead of myself and letting out secrets about our survival. I find on Ebay a job lot of e-chart cartridges which should fit the old chart plotter and cover the mid-Atlantic islands – the Azores, the Canaries and even some of the Caribbean in case we get washed right around the bath. You're not supposed to rely on electronic charts but buying enough paper to be sure we have the right set of islands is daunting. If I think better of it, we'll buy paper charts in Newport. The world centre of yachting must have charts. Buying charts always feels like hubris to me, the assumption being that you're going to arrive.

The Texan wind vane owner enjoyed his daughter's graduation and has forgivingly taken my much delayed Paypal payment and insured and dispatched the wind vane to Connecticut. It should be about a week in transit, and it has all sorts of little extra bits like a spares kit, spare specialist minimum-stretch control line, and pulleys. I have to get two 'top-tubes' because those are slightly different for a Cardinal than for the Island Packet to which the vane was previously fitted. I had phoned up the manufacturer in California before buying which turned out to be one of the most delightful companies I have ever dealt with. In return for the serial number of the vane, they could tell me immediately that the age I had been given was correct, and that they had installation drawings for a Cardinal 47 which means that they could bend two top-tubes if and when.

Does a Cardinal 47 have the same stern as a Cardinal 46? I google for a 47 but, apart from a good deal of ecclesiastical history, I can find nothing. I google the email for the designer, Alan Warwick, and explain I've just bought a 46 and ask him if it's the same as his 47. He very kindly emails back by return to say that if there is a Cardinal 47 out there, it's nothing to do with him. Probably a typo in the wind vane database. So I get a fax of the installation diagram and a quote for top-tubes.

I play little part in the major game of equipping because I lack the skills, or rather I do it at my own more domestic level which consists of lists of clothing for all weathers, medical supplies and prescription drugs, bathroom necessities like soap and our electric toothbrushes, kitchen equipment like sharp knives and a baking tin for bread. I devise menus. I book an appointment with my GP and persuade him to hand over local anaesthetic, dressings for burns, needles and thread for stitching flesh and heavy duty drugs for pain and tropical illnesses. He asks who is going to stitch serious wounds and cope with burns and fractures and I say Me. He looks bemused but gives me a very fast lesson on Accident and Emergencies.

This is very theoretical and unreal but I try to imagine not being able to pop out to Tesco or Boots or anywhere else for up to four weeks. I need novels. I need music. I need a good pillow. Stefan won't worry about creature comforts. He has more important things to think about and anyway, he is more or less oblivious to his surroundings. As long as the boat is sailing nicely, he will be content.

In the meantime we begin the name game, which becomes a constant background refrain. Very tiring after a while:

'Blue' (colour of hull, cherished film);

'Claudia' (Cardinale, but also 'was the weather');

'Scarlett' (O'Hara, American gal, Hawthorne's 'Scarlet Letter'). Good name for a blue boat. Everyone likes Scarlett though there is some agonising over the number of ts, one of which eventually gets lost in applying to the Small Ships Register.

Engine spares next. The engine is a 55 hp converted VW Rabbit, some sort of US version of a Polo engine, which apparently has a genuine 250 hours on it. Two thousand hours would be low for the age of boat. But this isn't necessarily good news. Lying in a seawater-damp bilge unused for long periods isn't the best way of life for a diesel. I phone up the company who converted the engine in Canada and ask them what they would advise given these circumstances. They recommend I change the timing belt because they perish, and if they go, the valves get damaged. I order spare fan and alternator belts too, and a spare marine alternator (ouch!) and some gasket sets which are recommended for emergencies. Another helpful small company.

Electricity is complicated for Europeans on a US boat with two voltages and different frequencies. For example, we have a laptop for displaying planning charts, so we need either an inverter to produce 240 volts AC, or a 12V adaptor to run straight from the batteries. Scarlet has an inverter which produces 115 volts AC from battery power. In the end we decide on the DC adapter. Same with a battery charger to charge dry batteries for Gecko. And a large box of batteries – dry cells to Americans. I have an inbuilt horror of depending on juice we don't have.

Communications next. There's a single sideband radio on the boat's inventory which will pick up weather faxes, forecasts, and cruiser networks, and which has an email modem which should connect to the laptop for outward email. We have a backup Sony world band pocket radio which also picks up SSB, and runs on dry batteries independent of the ship's electrics. I've never used a SSB, though I have all the tickets for GMDSS short range (VHF) operations, if I can remember any of it. I'm not much keener on ships' radios than the phone. There are legion family stories about my devious ways of getting others to operate the VHF. The first mate, in contrast, has a full, long distance, short wave radio operator's certificate required for the SSB. I was too busy to go on that particular course at the last minute. If, dear reader, you find all this technical stuff horribly detailed, bewildering and boring, so do we, but without it we could never capture the essential flavour of the mental processes of preparing for this trip.

Hmm. Radio operator's certificate! Guess who was sent down to Southampton at this point for a three day Communications Course? Stefan decided it would be a good idea, as well as a legal requirement, if one of us could use the VHF and the Single Sideband and knew what to do with the EPERB and somehow I drew the short straw but the real reason for sending me instead of going himself was his hatred of phones which includes speaking into a VHF. He'll do anything not to pick up the mic.

I did the most basic sailing course – Competent Crew – a good few years ago, taught by a hardened sailor whose refrain to the three women enrolled was: 'You'll be busy in the galley so I don't know why you are on this course.' In my case, he was probably right. I have to squeeze my brain very hard to grasp even the most fundamental rules of navigation and the pathetic few facts I retained for the exam, fell out the minute the course finished.

So there I was in a seedy B & B, in a single bedroom that was obviously half a previous room, with noisy pipes and wallpaper that offended my sensibilities. There were four of us on the course. A supremely confident middle-aged woman who ran her own business and had just bought a brand new boat with all the trimmings for racing and blue water cruising. She knew what she was doing. Her brand new Land Rover was full of gadgets and she gave me my first introduction to a Tom Tom. Back then, they weren't so common. She was formidable and established early on that there would be no jokes about women skippers. One of the two men, always in his business suit and often exiting to take calls on one of his three mobiles, owned an eighty-six foot ice-breaker. No lack of funds there either. The second man had been sent on the course by his company and stayed fairly quiet. All three were perfectly capable already and were doing the course only as a formality. I was the dunce. The teacher was relaxed and funny, and knew his stuff. For three long days we took copious notes about all kinds of equipment and how it worked. Wave bands and radio waves and satellites and safety routines. We practised emergency calls to and from the coast guard (the teacher), telling him were sinking/on fire/crushed by a super-tanker/had spotted three men in the water, and sent urgent messages to one another, always using the correct protocol. I tried to learn endless variations of Mayday! Mayday! Ice-breaker-Man and I were in the same lodgings so in the evenings we sat in the migraine-carpeted lounge while he tried to explain what I had not grasped. He was very patient.

The exam was in three parts. First, a written paper supervised by an external examiner. Then a series of mock scenes in which the examiner played the coastguard and we were skippers in distress. The third part was a practical exam using all the mock equipment. By this stage, the teacher had grasped I was a hopeless case and advised the others to go first in the mock communications and told me to try to remember what they had said. When I totally failed the mock written exam, he suggested I cheat by sitting close to Ice-Breaker-Man and copying his answers. Well, the other three passed. Land Rover Woman didn't drop a single mark. I was called back into the room to face the examiner who said I had failed but he would give me a second chance. Bless them, they didn't like to fail people who had paid £350 to become competent. I managed to answer his questions – but everyone knew it was a stitch-up.

It became a running joke on our ocean crossing that I was the communications expert. I had the certificate to prove it.

Clothing? Just how warm, hot, cold will it be wherever it is we turn out to be? I have a lightish grade breathable anorak and dungarees, and I think this is a good medium bet. With several pullovers underneath it ought to be good for any cold we're likely to meet and may be more than is needed, with luck. But my experience of nights at sea is that it gets cold even when it's warm. Lynn has a good anorak but needs waterproof trousers, and Louis needs a full suit. We decide to buy in Connecticut, bearing in mind what can be carried onto the plane. Turning up for the flight in full heavy-weather gear might prove tricky. We have a daunting shopping list for the last minute – flares, tools, fixings, useful bits and pieces, in fact all the stuff that you collect in Tupperware boxes when you own a boat and go cruising, but don't collect when your boat is parked at the yacht club.

Louis keeps threatening fishing. I can't tell quite whether he is winding up his Mamma or deadly serious. He obsesses about fishing gear out of all proportion to the vital not-yet-done-jobs-on-which-our-lives-will-depend. It's nearly as out of proportion as my Ebay searching. There's possibly an element of displacement activity on both our parts?

When I read people's accounts of their preparations for voyages I see that they take three months off work, put their new boats through their paces, stow, re-stow and label, and then redesign the rig, and so on. I console myself that Robin Knox-Johnson set off and spent the first week diving over the side to stuff caulking cotton into a leaking seam. But then I remember that he was a professional, and had sailed that particular boat back from India first.

Which brings us to our degree of experience. I have been sailing dinghies since I was seven, starting with Dad on the river, and towing the boat to the seaside some summer holidays. At nine I made a fatal trip with Dad to the London boat show and still vividly remember being spellbound by what must have been a 35 foot wooden sailing cruiser in the cavern of Earl's Court. We queued for two hours and the laminated oak frames and varnished mahogany planking are still engraved in my memory, along with the smell of a newly varnished wooden boat. After that, I took up residence in the bottom of my father's wardrobe, where he kept his sailing books. I planned my ocean voyaging, curled up in the wardrobe bottom, lost to the world and my mother. I can still minutely visualise the diagrams of Peter Heaton's ideal cruising boat, and the salty pictures of the gaffer's bow-wave among the photos in the middle pages of the book.

⚓

CHAPTER 8

Past experience

Apart from sporadic dinghy sailing with my father, that was it, until Lynn and I got married and bought a 24 footer we kept on the Mersey mud and sailed around the Welsh coast. Baptism by water! The whole coast is without refuge from when the tide is half-out until it is half in again, and whenever we went near the boat, it blew something wicked. We have rather too-vivid memories of surfing over the Menai Straits bar in a huge following Atlantic sea, and wondering whether we had the channel lined up exactly right. We got bar-bumping down to a fine art.

Finally we got caught out by a July force nine several hours ahead of its Met Office cue. It came out of nowhere and caught us waiting for the last six inches of tide to reach refuge. A rescue helicopter turned up spontaneously, and, with a small son on board, discretion was the better part of valour. The pilot admitted after they had been called out to a separate distress call and happened to see us on the way back, and didn't fancy having their lunch disturbed a second time. The boat broke her anchor chain a few hours later and was splintered on the rocks.

What! That's not how I remember it. 'A rescue helicopter turned up spontaneously . . .' This is not mere understatement but the transformation of reality after the event. This is what actually happened.

A couple of friends had come down to stay with us and go for a sail. Tim had never sailed before so this was to be his maiden voyage. The weather was looking a bit unsettled by the time we all reached the beach but Stef said it was nothing to worry about. He dragged the small inflatable from where we kept it tied to a rock and rowed off with small son Adam and Tim on board while Sally and I watched and waited from the shore. Louis was very young. Even as they rowed, the waves became choppy and the sky darkened. It began to look like very hard work. About half way out we could see Stef pulling hard on the oars with very little effect. It took a long, long time for them to reach the boat which by now was tossing its head as high a horse trying to get out of its halter. Up it rose, pulling the anchor chain tight, then down it fell into the waves. Up and down. Sally and I could make out the three figures on deck and behind them we could see the storm clouds gathering. Then one figure on deck. Stef. The others must have gone below. By now, other people had walked down to the beach and were watching with us. Some had binoculars. Our small boat continued to toss and strain. Sally and I paced up and down the beach, me carrying Louis. Someone said that it wasn't safe to be on that boat. A man came up to us and said that he was really worried and asked if we wanted him to call out the rescue helicopter. Sally and I both nodded. Another woman, now at our side, said she had already called. I think several people had. It was on its way.

Once the helicopter was hovering over the boat, Sally and I thought all would now be well. But what was this? My husband looked like he was waving his arms as if to shoo the helicopter away. What!

'I want my husband off there.' Sally said. Her face was grim.

'I want my son off.' I agreed.

'What the hell is he doing?' Sally asked, as the helicopter whirred away and landed on the beach.

'What's happening?' we yelled, when it was safe to run underneath the blades.

'The skipper won't come off. Says he'll be OK.'

What!

'It's not safe . . .' I started to say.

'Nothing we can do if the skipper refuses to leave his boat though I agree he's not safe out there in this wind and in these sea conditions. The anchor chain could break.'

'Go back and get my son!' I shouted. 'I want my son off that boat.'

'And my husband!' Sally yelled above the noise of the blades.

The yellow bird flew again and there was Stef waving his long arms in a No Thank You gesture while clinging to the rails to stop himself being tossed overboard. His clothes streamed out horizontally in the gale. But this time as the helicopter hovered above the boat, a rope was thrown out, and one of the rescue men climbed down it. The sky was so dark it was hard to see anything from the shore, but when the rescue man next appeared on the rope, he had a small person with him. Thank God. My son reached the helicopter safely and was taken inside. The valiant rescue man climbed down again and this time Tim was hoisted with him. Back came the helicopter and Sally and I raced to it, both weeping with relief.

And Stef?

'Still wants to stay with the boat.'

By now most of the villagers and holiday makers were on the sand, watching the adventure. The wind was so ferocious, it was hard to stay upright. All of us watched the boat rise, strain and fall. Rise and fall. The creaking of the anchor chain could be heard across the water.

'We'll go back and get him off,' one of the men said. 'This is a Force 8. The boat is going to break its chain any minute.'

Back they went a third time. Stef was persuaded off, and I turned a deaf ear to his curses when he was put down on the beach. Minutes later the chain broke and she was carried across the bay as helpless as a paper boat. She was hurled on to rocks. There she crashed and splintered.

The next morning, we stood on the sand dunes above the rocks and looked down on our broken boat. She was on her side and smashed beyond repair. The waves, calmer than the previous day, washed over her.

I took yacht master classes as a penance.

*

Lynn is a sunshine person so next we bought a sixth share of a 33' cruiser in Mallorca, and spent every holiday with the kids going from beach to beach and enjoying all the places you can only get to by boat. In Mallorca the problem was usually too little wind rather than too much, though there were a couple of interesting escapades. Such fond memories. Louis, aged about three, sitting in the cool box full of sea water eating watermelon in about 105 degrees of heat while I tried to coax the oil spill out of the engine bilge with a thimble. This sort of family sailing doesn't put on the night hours, or do much for the navigational skills. I did the theory courses, astro in those days, and a one week practical course, sailing off Oban. So I had all the tickets and a fair amount of sailing experience, but was woefully lacking in the long distance department. Lynn ditto. Louis first went sailing on the Welsh coast when two weeks old, rowed out to the boat in his carry cot, balanced on Mum's knees. So it was in the blood, but his long distance experience was even less than mine.

Then in the 1980s the family got ill. Very ill. We spent, on and off, fifteen years struggling with Lynn and Louis recovering and relapsing from ME. Housebound. Bedbound. Learning to live with and manage a severe chronic illness that was not understood. We sold the boat share and gave up sailing. There was one charter fortnight in Turkey during a rare interlude when they were both a bit better. But Lynn was fairly bad on the boat, and one afternoon when she had passed out, and I was more than a bit sleepy, I very nearly put our Turkish-flagged boat into a nearby Greek harbour. Confidently sailing towards what I thought was a Turkish island, I noticed a destroyer displaying a Greek flag anchored a short distance off shore. "Must be practising their deceptions," my overheated brain thought. But it didn't quite compile, and I did a uey smart.

We finally escaped the ME ghetto. I can't go back there. I don't like to write about it. I'm frightened to tempt fate. It was 1987 when we all got flu and didn't get better. There were seven of us affected by the same virus, all from or linked to Stefan's academic department, including the very fit American head of department, the Irish administrator, a lecturer and a couple of the post-docs. And my two sons and me. It took between three and twenty years for us to recover.

Louis was the most severely affected, but not initially. His was a more gradual onset. He struggled through alternate years at primary school, pale and exhausted, but when he started secondary school, he completely crashed. The input and effort was an overload for someone as sick as he was. That was pretty much the end of his schooling. From the age of 13, he spent four years in bed – and I mean in bed, not getting up, not doing anything. We were living outside Edinburgh in a small claustrophobic village and he could see the other kids playing football from his window. He was incredibly stoic. Louis became ill when he was six. He is thirty now, married, and working as a photographer, but certainly not fit. Firing on two cylinders but always managing his energy.

After seven years I felt well enough to go back to work, tempted by an attractive research grant and a base in a very good research department in Glasgow. But it meant commuting from Edinburgh and often staying overnight. Big mistake. Eighteen months later, I was back in bed. The relapse was worse than the initial onset of the illness and that was the end of sailing for a few years.

But I have fond memories of those first holidays in Mallorca, before Louis caved in and I relapsed. The boys grew up with the sea as their playground. Louis was a water-baby from early on and could only be coaxed from playing in the water when the sun was setting and his fingers were totally wrinkled. I remember a very small Adam, before Louis was born, sitting in the prow of our first twenty footer, so padded by his life-jacket that his arms stuck out sideways, chanting like a mantra, 'Another wave; another wave; another wave . . .' until his head lolled sideways and we knew he had fallen asleep. I remember Louis sitting in the cold-box with a grin the same shape as his slice of watermelon. Both boys were at home on the boat and in the water. They fished and surf-boarded and swam and drove around bays and harbours in the dinghy and went crabbing with nets. I am a confident swimmer and have respect but not fear of the sea. Perhaps they picked up my enthusiasm and delight. We were all of us very at home on our scruffy old Moody, but Louis's enthusiasm for boats was inbuilt and enduring. Like father, like son.

But as Stef says, with two boys on board, we mostly pottered from cove to cove, rarely doing more than three hours' sailing at a stretch, and then with the coast always in sight. A lot of time was spent anchored in magic, hidden places, accessible only by sea. The sailing was secondary to the playing. We lived in a caravan on water.

Finally, finally, Lynn's health got a bit better, and we chartered a boat – just the two of us – because by now our son was grown up though still ill. We sailed around the Saronics. Fantastic! We were coming back to life. The next two years' holidays were spent on a one-fifth share of a new Bavaria 38 based in Croatia. There was wind, more than we had been used to, and we managed some nighttime shenanigans each time the anchor was blown out of the thin sand by the Borra. But we only had limited offshore experience.

So here we were, about to fly to the US to sail Scarlet back across the pond when the farthest we'd been from land was about 20 miles. Lots of experience interacting with coasts! Very little with oceans. Or boatyards.

CHAPTER 9

⚓

Hiccups

MAY 2005

I absolutely can't be out of the office before 31st May. Non-negotiable. This means we can sea trial Scarlet with the surveyor on 1st June. One week's hard coastal sailing to flush out the problems and get our sea legs. I'm always very wary of getting out of the office and straight onto a boat, yet there is usually incredible pressure to do just that, because holiday time is so limited. But I just know that I'm useless going straight from my desk on to a boat. There's usually been some crisis and I really ought to go to bed in a darkened room for a week, or just lie in the sun. There's something about office mentality and sailing mentality which are deeply incompatible. But here we are about to be sandwiched up against hurricane season. We're supposed to be out of Bermuda by early June. It is just about possible, and we can always duck out and go back to the US and spend the holiday spuddling about getting to know our new boat, which is exactly what we should be doing anyway. That's what all the books say.

Oh, you ask, how long is our holiday? And how long does it take to sail to the Canaries from Newport, RI? Well, to take the second question first, it's about 2,300 nautical miles and if one were to average about 100 miles a day – about 4 knots – then it would take 23 days, wouldn't it? Scarlet should do much better than that. We have four weeks holiday so we should be back in time – a simple calculation.

Crew number estimation is more complex. Our third member of the crew, our son Louis, has a newish girlfriend, Iona, and their plans seem undecided:

1. Iona is going to fly with Louis to California where they will visit her friend Murdo. Then Louis will come down to Connecticut alone and take ship;
2. Iona is going to fly with Louis to New York, and then both of them will join us in Connecticut where they will help us prepare the boat before Iona flies alone to California to visit her friend Murdo;
3. Ditto above except during preparation time Iona will persuade Louis to go with her to California to visit Murdo instead of risking his life crossing the ocean with his mad parents.

Lynn and I thought that we had all agreed on Option 1, but as it turned out later, Option 3 remained an ongoing, nerve-racking possibility. This last permutation would be a serious problem. Our insurance won't cover us transatlantic for a crew of two because insurers sensibly don't like small crews. So if Louis didn't come, we couldn't come either.

And so we all walked an extra emotional tightrope for the few weeks before voyage time. This tightrope walk seemed to cover the full length of the rope in both directions, several times.

But I'm getting ahead of myself. This part of the story must wait until later. However it is relevant because I have to buy charts, and before I buy charts, it would be helpful to know where we will be sailing. I opt for the worst case scenario – a cruise in the Chesapeake for two. To forestall this eventuality really happening, I buy a cruising guide to the Chesapeake. In fact so concerned am I about being short-crewed and not allowed to cross the pond (even spuddling in the Chesapeake, I would very much value having Louis's wisdom, muscle and company) that I buy *two* cruising guides to the Chesapeake. Normally one is enough to guarantee we will wind up elsewhere, but this calls for double strength precautions. While buying them on the web, I find out that we aliens are not allowed to buy charts of the US since 9/11. Or rather, I think I have bought them on the web. I have certainly paid for them on the web. But then an email informs me that they cannot, by Federal Law, be posted to their new owner, and no I can't have a refund.

One more hiccup. We find out by accident that the insurance company has not received the copy of the survey I faxed them, so the boat is only insured for inside the shed. I sent the survey off, and it failed to arrive, and I forgot that I hadn't heard from them. Because the survey was so obviously OK, it just slipped my mind that we hadn't heard the insurance company say that it was OK. Good job we found out in time. We fax them the surveyor's report.

A further sub-hiccup.

'Sorry we can't insure you because the standing rigging (useful stuff that holds the mast up) is more than 12 years old.'

Apparently, there is no such thing as a survey that will satisfy these insurers about rigging that is more than 12 years old. I express gratitude that they have waited until now to tell me this.

'We didn't have the survey,' they say in their defense.

The survey says the rigging is fine, and says nothing about the age of the rigging.

'But the rigging is more than twelve years old.'

Which was on the form we originally filled in months ago. So the boat is uninsured for sailing. It's OK tied to the dock, or for motoring across the Atlantic with the mast down on the deck.

The 31st May flight is getting nearer. The surveyor, boatyard and broker are all lined up for 1st June, which is immediately after Memorial Day weekend when all the local boats will have been put in the water and the yard can concentrate on us. Yes, the yard will have it in the water. The life raft has been bought on Ebay in upstate New York and shipped to a servicer just up the road from the boatyard who promises it will be ready before the 1st. The dinghy and outboard are on their way and, courtesy of the delights of our electronic age, we can track them to a warehouse in Philadelphia where they arrived a mere thirty-six hours after dispatch from a secret origin. The EPIRB, also found new but shop soiled on Ebay, has arrived at the boatyard already, as have the paper charts. We get the EPIRB number from the seller so we can register it.

Buying an EPIRB means that it has to be registered with some authority who will take an interest when it goes off. There are chilling stories of sailors being lost because their EPIRB was unregistered. My antennae are highly sensitised to the word 'registration,' by now, but I am pleasantly surprised that there is a form on the web, and I post it off to Cornwall with the 16 digit EPIRB registration number. I have the second-hand e-charts with me because the seller happened to live in London.

This is unreal. The idea that we own a 46 ft sailing boat and are about to sail across the Atlantic is totally unreal. But then it *is* unreal because as things stand we will actually be going cruising in the Chesapeake, and then only under motor with the mast on deck. I read the cruising guide and I learn about the prevalence of jellyfish in the Chesapeake. The first mate combines a seriousness about her swimming with an intense distaste for jellyfish. In Croatia, after a good long swim away from the boat, she had just placed a first foot on the ladder when she screamed. Afterwards, she said that it was as if she had been stabbed with a knife and the first few minutes as she pulled herself aboard were pure agony. Later her thigh swelled and a deep ache continued for days. Once bitten, twice shy.

Now we have to get off the internet and across the Atlantic eastwards. All our gear is packed, and if our plane squeaks over the fence at the end of the runway it'll be doing well with this weight on board.

CHAPTER 10

Functions

31 MAY 2005

We arrive in the boatyard after a six-hour flight and four-hour drive, just before dusk, in a really violent thunderstorm. Sympathetic weather? A warning shot from the Gods? Very unusual weather, we are told later.

During the drive, in my feverish imagination, I am already down below staring in disbelief at this beautiful boat which is ours. I am making up the bunks for our first night aboard. Unfolding duvet covers and patting pillows, heating soup and buttering crusty bread. I will light candles when we snuggle down for the first time.

So heavy is the rain that we cannot see our boat although it is somewhere out there in the water about ten yards ahead. Nor can we get out of the car. After an hour peering through the streaming windscreen, the rain thins a bit, a rainbow arches across the sky, and we think that we can make out a familiar Cardinal-like shape.

Except that there is no mast.

No rigging.

No sails.

Literally a bare boat.

Can't be ours. Can it?

We jump out of the car into basin-like puddles and rain that hurts, and run to the boat. It's ours. But it's locked. Why haven't they left it open? They knew we were coming. Both companionways (yes, there are two) are closed with those padlocks of a thousand number combinations. What to do? We crawl all over her, peer in, and then settle in the monsoon to work our way through every number from 0000 onwards. Twice. At last we break in.

What has happened to the shiny interior we saw at Christmas? The polished galley? The arrangement of artificial flowers?

The floorboards are up.

The bilges are exposed.

The engine locker is open with parts spilling out.

There is no bedding. There isn't a bunk free of a ton of sails, anchors, bits of rigging, power tools and WD40.

I am breathing through squashed straws because my asthma has been triggered by all the dirt and dust but still I refuse to let go of my dream. We promised ourselves we would spend the first night on the boat alone, before our son and his girlfriend arrive tomorrow. Champagne and hugs. We can move stuff and still sleep here.

No, we can't.

We can.

We can't.

At 11 p.m. we set off for the Welcome Inn hoping they have a room. Hoping they are open.

Next morning, we breakfast on eggy bread, maple syrup and lots of coffee, with the toy train still going round and round its ledge below the ceiling carrying Christmas presents in its wagons.

We drive down to the boatyard, meet all the folks we've been pestering for weeks by phone and email, and get a good look at our boat. The mast is on trestles on the jetty. The surveyor turns up – a plausible chap – nor is he too bothered that we can't take her away from the jetty. Harness her well, and we can run the engine full throttle where she is. Everything else can be checked out right here, and the mast will get a better inspection than it would if it were up.

The surveyor starts his routine. First the infamous uninsurable standing rigging while it's lying down. He takes me over the mast and its fittings and the rod rigging. It looks good to me, and I sigh a large sigh of relief that it looks good to him. I explain about the insurance company, and he clearly regards their position as out of line. The broker offers to put me in touch with his buddy, Morgan, who will fix me up with insurance. The first of many calls to Morgan is put through.

The survey continues. He checks the engine belt tensions and the oil level, starts the engine, checks that the cooling water is flowing out of the transom (reassuringly loudly), checks the oil pressure and the sight glasses for the diesel filters. He warms up the engine and leaves it to run for a minute, then revs it up in neutral to check the smoke colour. He tells me these engines are not his favourite. Apparently the stainless exhausts corrode inside from the lack of air, and the *vorsprung durch teknik* has the water temperature running just short of boiling, which he feels is verging on the un-American. But the 250 hours on the clock looks as if it may be genuine. He puts the engine in gear at lowish revs and I watch the dock lines while he squeezes up the power. The dock lines strain, but the engine sounds good, and the cooling water is really gushing out of the stern pipe, which is nice and visible, and better still, noisy. That will save cricked necks peering over the transom. We have 80 amps coming out of the alternator and going into the batteries. He shows me how to read the battery monitoring system, a hive of functions. Taking up the floorboards, he listens to the prop shaft and the gearbox. Not so happy. A slight ticking noise, and the gear shift is both sticky and a little noisy. Not something I'd have picked up on an unfamiliar boat.

He runs me through the other thousand functions of the electronics – chart plotter 1, chart plotter 2, radar, log, depth, speed, VHF, and on and on. We go through the forty switches on the panel. A lot of the gear is subtly different from its European counterpart, or it is stuff I've never had, and all the terms are different. I'm as anti-function as I am anti-phone. On most of the few gadgets I possess, I only use the on-off switch, and the station they are tuned to when I buy them is the station they stay tuned to until they break. I was hoping that Louis would help with this function overload. He laps up functions in a way utterly incomprehensible to me. It reminds me of my father who was an electronic engineer who *designed* functions, and still rarely used them himself, and is probably some obscure part of the reason I can't deal with them. The idea that I'm going to be able to use any of this stuff while bobbing about feeling green is quite fanciful.

The fridge and freezer are running off dock power – one of the first things Lynn checked as she likes her beer cold. The surveyor turns them off and engages the engine-driven compressor to make sure they will work at sea. The compressor is a horrendous great beast at the front of the engine which audibly slows the 55 hp diesel when it is engaged. But the fridge seems to be working. White frost appears on its metal connector to the black rubber pipe so something is getting cold.

The surveyor shows me how to work the radar – a piece of equipment I am totally unfamiliar with but one that is rather important in the fog generated by the Labrador Current off this east coast. He has to poke a lot of buttons because he's unfamiliar with this particular model, but once he figures it out, he goes on to show me which ones are essential to its proper care and feeding. More function indigestion. We finally get a green image of the boatyard shed. I suppose if a forty foot high tin shed doesn't show up it really isn't working. Whether the converse holds …

We have a good look at the bilges, pumps and seacocks and stuff. We flush the two heads. We test the pressurised water and the manual fresh and salt water pumps. All the rest of the boat he surveyed in the shed back in February. He pronounces himself happy except for the gearbox/clutch mechanism and its subtle mysterious noise. The broker agrees that it will have to come out and be checked over. Bill from the boatyard starts right in. The surveyor and broker head home.

The mast, in the meantime, is about to go up. It's craned to the vertical and swung over until Pete catches the bottom and Fred helps him drop it through the hole in her deck. It's a keel-stepped mast that sits on the keel, rather than on deck. The forestay has roller furling, the shrouds and the backstay, infamous standing rigging, are joined to the deck and bottle-screwed tight. These are two very experienced riggers and they are only too keen to find problems. They say the rigging is good; that if it had been up for fifteen years without attention, then they might have to agree with the insurance people, but this rigging has been disassembled every year. The trouble starts with corrosion around the fittings, but if they are undone every year, inspected, and lubricated, they are reliable. Racing is the other concern because perfectly uncorroded rigging could still be over-stressed and work-hardened, but that doesn't seem likely given how little the boat has been used. I get on to Morgan, the insurance broker, faxing him a record of our experience and qualifications, explaining the intended itinerary, value and age of the boat and so on. He thinks that it may be better to find insurance at Lloyd's in London rather than on the US market since the Canaries, our most likely first stop, are European. He says that refusing rigging merely on age grounds is unusual and he doesn't *think* there'll be a problem.

Meanwhile, Lynn has been mucking out. The boat is absolutely filthy, full of dust from the sanding and spraying jobs that go on in the shed in the winter months. She has been going at it like a demented badger digging its set with clouds of dirt flying out along with complaints about boats that haven't been cleaned for twenty years. She wears dirty cargoes and pink rubber gloves.

When there is enough space for us to lie down, we begin to feel our aches and pains and decide to call it a day. The jet lag is beginning to take hold. A sandwich from the deli, a shower under the marina hose (it's about 85 degrees outside at 8.00 p.m.) and we collapse on the captain's bunk.

It is our first night aboard Scarlet but no champagne corks are popping. We are too knackered to celebrate.

CHAPTER 11

⚓

A rusty water tank

JUNE 2005

Rise and shine with the dawn jet lag rota. The jetty has moved up about a couple of meters with the ebb tide. I go in search of orange juice and muffins for breakfast. I discover a charming New England village, American flags stuck in manicured lawns, up-market tourist clothes shops, all intensely leafy now that the ice we saw in February has melted.

Back at the boat, I turn on the galley tap and it spits a bit of rusty water at me. That's very odd. I filled the tanks yesterday from the dock hose. Probably just air bubbles locked in the pipes. More brown water spits out. Then pure air and somewhere down in the nether regions, the pump is whining. Where are the 150 gallons of water I put in the tanks yesterday evening? Well, they have to be in the bilge, don't they? I lift the floor panel above the deepest sump in the bilge. No water. At least, not 150 gallons. If there is a leak in the bilge, water comes in, it doesn't go out. That's the problem with boats isn't it? Well, maybe something is working: the automatic bilge pump? Come to think of it, there were noises last night that might have been a bilge pump. Amid the so many new noises – the fridge and freezer, the current under the jetty, the traffic on the river – I didn't pay much attention.

I meet Bill on my way to the office and he too is surprised we have no water. He takes a quick look and satisfies himself it's all gone. It's not that easy to check the tank levels but it transpires that Bill has been looking after the internal systems of this boat ever since it came to this yard, and if Bill says it's empty, then it's empty. But why?

He diagnoses for a few minutes before deciding that the problem is probably in the hot water circuit. The hot water tank heats off the engine, as well as off the mains electricity, and the hot tank is fed from the cold water tanks, so if the hot circuit is leaking, the whole system can empty. There are telltale damp rust marks draining into the bilge from where the hot tank sits in the bottom of the cavernous cockpit locker.

It's a good job that the tank didn't wait to empty itself until we were in the middle of the Atlantic. That would have been half our water gone. There is a second tank but we haven't turned it on yet. So what's the damage? And to whom? It's fairly major excavations to get to the empty hot tank to make sure that the diagnosis is correct and Bill starts immediately. An hour later there is a two-foot cube steel tank on the dockside with the entire bottom rusted out.

As far as I am concerned this is the owner's lookout; it's a defect that couldn't be checked in a freezing shed in midwinter so it's covered by the escrow. I phone the broker and he agrees. How long is it going to take to get a replacement tank? It has to be very similar in size and shape to fit into the existing space and to allow a join with the pipe labyrinth – input water, output water, engine coil in, engine coil out, winter drain tap, electric supply for the immersion heater, earth (sorry 'ground'). Systems! So many systems! Al, the foreman, gets on the phone to hunt tanks.

Lynn and I have breakfast: coffee, orange juice and muffins. Very restorative! We lean back in the cockpit and drink it all in for the first time. She really is magnificent. What a form! So beautifully thought out and constructed. The mast goes up and up and up for ever and just as we're admiring it, Pete the rigger comes by. He too glances upwards. Then down at the ground. He looks nervous. He doesn't look me in the eye.

'Er . . . did you guys notice . . . er . . .'

It's clear he is not quite sure whether to ask this next question.

'I would say there's no trickler on that masthead.'

Three heads crane upwards.

'I mean . . . if I were headed off across the pond . . . I don't think I'd do that without masthead navigation lights.'

He's right. There are no tricolour lights at the top of the never-ending mast. And I hadn't even noticed.

Pete is still looking squeamish as if he's not quite sure whether he ought to be pointing this out to the boat's owner. Judging owners must be a tricky but major occupational hazard.

The mast has been stepped in the boatyard without navigation lights. This (almost) owner saw that there was no tricolour on the masthead when the mast was down on its trestles on the jetty, but assumed that the fitting was yet to be plugged in, and was too busy worrying about the possibility of owning uninsurable standing rigging to pursue it. And so the mast went up unlit. Yes, we definitely ought to have a tricolour on top so that ships can see us, and I'm very grateful for being told about its absence. Pete relaxes, subtly. Strictly speaking, we are legal with the red and the green lights on the pulpit, but they're at best seven feet above the sea and therefore visible for about a mile if we're lucky. Not far enough. It seems a very unlikely omission from the inventory of a generally well-equipped yacht but then I am beginning to understand the implications of the previous owner's habit of day sailing. Occasionally.

Next thing Pete is being dangled from the masthead by Fred working at the winch, trying to see if he can access inside the masthead sheave-box ('shiv box' – love that word!) to get a supply cable down the mast. He has an endoscope – an optic fibre gizmo designed originally to satisfy medical curiosity about malfunctioning bowels – so that he can see what goes on inside the mast. Then he's down at the bottom of the mast doing the same to see how to get the wire out at the keel-step. He gets himself right side-up and announces that the news is not good. The mast is made with a baffle at the top and another at the bottom so that it's virtually impossible to thread a fish-wire and pull a cable through. The mast has to come out, and the shiv box off. He says he has done them before up at the top but it usually winds up even more expensive because of the time it takes. This needs an understanding with the office. Just what is the damage? This is my fault; a very expensive lapse of attention.

The day's plan, which we had discussed over breakfast before Pete dropped by with his bombshell observation, was for me to think about mounting the wind vane on the transom. The installation will have to wait until Louis arrives. The top-tubes have arrived from CA and the vane from TX. The cardboard box containing the wind vane box is five foot high and three foot square. I start unpacking like a small boy with a very large and much anticipated Christmas present. I am immediately submerged in a mound of polystyrene chips. Various bits of tube emerge. A vane here, a hydrofoil there, and then the main frame with the doings, all massive three-inch shiny stainless steel tubes with beautifully verdigris bronze pinion gears and bearings. Not to forget the book of words. This is such a beautiful piece of engineering; it radiates thoughtfulness and a few hundred thousand miles of testing. I spend a couple of happy hours tracing out the causalities and checking that I know how it goes together and that it's all there. It's love at first sight and my initial reaction will prove well founded in the weeks ahead of us.

By now we have office information about the mast. To extract it and fit it again, this time with the tricolour in place, is going to cost an arm and a leg. Would we like it done over the weekend at overtime rates of two arms and two legs? Before we can decline, it transpires that Pete and Fred, along with the other yard hands, haven't had a day off since March 1st because of the spring mania that grips the yachting industry with people like us trying to get into the water. No, we'll wait until Monday while Pete and Fred try to remember what their kids look like. It will give us a better run at the wind vane installation because taking the mast down means detaching the backstay which is right in the middle of our scene of operations on the handsome transom. Two teams playing two games on the same pitch.

Further information reveals that a hot-water tank has been located in upstate New York. It is stainless steel instead of rustable but it won't be here for a week.

An unusually sensible need to take stock grabs me. Maybe it's the shock of failing to observe a mast without lights. I decide we must update our list of problems and issues. My last call to the broker revealed that the inventory is still dynamic.

Before we came out, we were told that that there was no SSB radio, no storm jib, and no inner forestay. The broker has now provided a storm jib. We agreed with the broker that as compensation for the absent SSB, the owner will pay for new canvas on the two spray hoods, and provide a new bimini, all to be fitted before we arrive. Now, running backstays have emerged from the loft, but no inner forestay. And nothing is fitted.

The day after we arrived, the canvas man turned up to measure the bimini and dodger and to cut out plastic templates. But they wouldn't be done for a week. They need to be fitted on the frames the following week, and will then be unfitted and taken away again for final stitching. Three or four days later, they will be returned and permanently fitted.

No SSB radio means that we have no long range communications, but fortunately, before coming, we decided to buy, as a back-up, a simple cheap satellite email and weather report system to provide rudimentary email messages in both directions and weather faxes across the Atlantic. This system collects satellite data, and has be told to change satellite for the European data somewhere in mid-Atlantic. We need to alert the operating company to that imminent change before departure.

"Yes, sir, the required widget will be delivered to CT in three days, and fitting it is a matter of half a day."

From the plans, I measure the run of wire which will be needed to put the aerial on top of the radar mast at the stern of the boat and the connection into the laptop on the navigator's desk.

There is an email from my brother Paul about the EPIRB. Cornwall has decided that we have to register it in the US. Having found all this out over the web, my brother gives me the password for the website where I can check that all the details are OK and add the new SSR number.

Fred's departing shot on Friday evening is that we are going to fry this weekend. Oh, and by the way, there's a gale forecast with a ten per cent probability of tornadoes. All with a wry New England smile! It's already getting hot.

We also have an update on the ETA of the crew. Son Louis and girlfriend Iona will arrive by train from New York late afternoon today. It is late afternoon now, though whether it is today, I couldn't say. Lynn is still mucking out and doesn't want to break off. I jump in the car and head for where I vaguely remember the train station was back in February. We drove past it, I think, when we were exploring. It has moved. I search in vain for a pedestrian to ask. Silly me! There are no pedestrians in America. I drive into town, pass over some railroad tracks, and home in on the station. The train is just about to pull in on the other side. From the bridge I can see there is no Louis or Iona. I return to the boat. Several hours later, they turn up at the boatyard by taxi.

CHAPTER 12

⚓

Wind vane

JUNE 2005

Early on Saturday morning I'm back to the village shop for juice and blueberry muffins. I rise earlier than the other three so take my large brown paper bag and my small cappuccino for a walk down by the water. It's still relatively cool – middle eighties. The river is peaceful. She has seen men come and launch their boats before, and heard them arguing, and pays not a jot of interest.

By the time I get back, the others are up. We munch our muffins in the rapidly rising heat. Between mouthfuls, Louis and I discuss the coming installation. DIY is one of our best modes of interaction. Ever since, at three years old, he used to peer into a malfunctioning car engine and confidently pronounce: "It's that black bit there that's wrong, Daddy!" while reaching for a spanner to sort it out. As part of Louis's very long slow recovery from ME, we built a sailing dinghy in the garage so he's quite a shipwright by now.

Scarlet's transom at present has her previous, highly objectionable, name SCRAP emblazoned in gold leaf, with NY, NY beneath. Fancy letters. Lousy name. We'll try to work around it.

Before we begin on the wind vane we need to arrange some shade. The telegraph-pole legs that hold up the jetty are at least eight feet high so we should be able to rig a line from the radar post on our starboard quarter to the nearest jetty post, to support a patchwork of tarpaulins that we have salvaged from behind the shed. That should keep off the worst of the midday sun, as long as we remember to keep adjusting for the tidal rise and fall.

We fasten the inflatable dinghy under Scarlet's stern so that one of us can work from the dinghy while the other works from the cockpit. The exact level of difficulty of the job will be determined by how accessible the inside of the transom is for holding the nuts firmly while I tighten the bolts that hold the four feet of the vane from the outside. If we (Louis) can't get into the lazarette – the deep but narrow locker that goes way down into the transom – then there's no way of doing it. No wind vane, no crossing.

When I bought the vane, I asked the guy at the manufacturers how difficult the installation would be. He told me that it depended on what the boat designer had put in the way, and how good a supply of small boys was available on the dock to be persuaded inside the locker, adding hastily that the tradition was to offer a dollar for each nut held on from inside while it is tightened up from outside. Looking around, I see no small boys on the dock, but initial excavations into the lazarette yield a ton of dock lines of various vintage, and the good news that there is a bit of space between the gas-locker and the transom. It looks as if Louis's physique will come into its own. Louis is of the linear ectomorph persuasion. If we oil him well and slide him head first into the starboard lazarette he should be able to reach the nuts for all four feet of the vane – two self locking nuts onto two bolts for each leg. It is pushing 105 degrees in the lazarette.

So we set to work. First we improvise a gantry to dangle this enormously heavy, gangly piece of apparatus over the transom to take the weight while we get it aligned. The vane has to be absolutely level, and within an inch of the right depth in the water or it will either dig itself in, or pull out, as the boat heels. The transom is sloped and curved and there is no right angle in sight, but we manage to find the midline and soon get the four metal struts and their feet sitting on the transom, much as should be with the height about right. There are two torsional struts which we never do manage to find room to fit, but we take comfort that the manual says they are a retrofit, and not strictly necessary.

Out with the newly bought battery drill and soon the transom of our shiny new boat is riddled with half-inch holes. The bolts go through a doddle, not forgetting the shake-proof washers. Still not a small boy in sight, so it's time to stow Louis in the lazarette. The muffled exclamations as he is fed in are painful to the paternal ear, but not nearly as painful as being fed in would be for the paternal midriff. Even he barely makes it – in both senses of the word bare. Consulting the tables at the back of the Encyclopedia of the Physiology of Extreme DIY, we calculate he has about two minutes forty-eight seconds to get his cramped fingers around the eight nuts to tighten them up before he runs out of oxygen. That's thirty-one seconds a nut. I descend into the dinghy and ratchet the nuts frantically. Eight done with seven and a half seconds to spare.

I am amused to find that the dinghy has moved around slightly so that the cooling water from the freezer that shoots out of the bottom of the transom has been filling it up as I work. I wondered why I had that rising damp sensation. Louis extracts himself and emerges half a stone skinnier – not previously thought possible – but still showing signs of life.

It's about two o'clock and the thermometer in the shade of the shed is registering 100 degrees. Humidity much the same. The lazarette must now be about 120 degrees. The remaining bits and pieces of the wind vane go on quickly until we are left with the last problem of running the special stretch resistant control lines back along one side of the cockpit, round a pulley and onto another pulley which is fixed to the boat's steering wheel. That's not a job for today. This afternoon we're going up the creek to find somewhere to wallow among the hippopotami.

The four of us set off with a picnic in the inflatable. The outboard starts right out of the box, and we're off, through the docks, past the jetties until the creek widens out into a reed encircled marsh. We run aground in six inches of water, about three hundred yards from land. We have to get out and push, but we're soon afloat again and then up on a little beach with a gully going through to the deeper water of the main channel.

Stripped off, we sit in the cool ooze up to our necks. The water is startlingly cold because it is still only just June and the last of the snow melt from the interior is still making its way to the sea. What a climate! Spring had not really arrived before we left the far north. The heat here is instantly relaxing, even the torrid humidity, provided that you are not stuffed into a lazarette, and as long as you don't have to read instructions, make plans or install a wind vane.

It's only when we stop that the full unreality hits. Here we are with just our heads poking out of some muddy water on a foreign continent 3000 miles from home having foresworn all normal methods of transport to get back. This is practically the first time we've drawn breath since we came. Louis and Iona disappear while Lynn and I sit on the beach. We don't need to say anything but we know that each is finding it difficult to believe that this is happening.

CHAPTER 13

A boat called Scrap

JUNE 2005

Next day, back at the boatyard, the owner turns up with an anchor and his wife in tow. The missing second anchor turns out to be folded up in the brown cardboard box in the bottom of the locker in the forepeak. The extra jib has been found, and two running-backs, but no inner-forestay. He accuses the yard of having the latter in their loft. Afterwards, Pete says discreetly that there never was an inner forestay. A new one has to be ordered from the local rigger who arrives to measure up, and is very thorough, observing that the foredeck fitting is obsolete and it wasn't properly backed by a plate. The whole purpose is to give some extra support to the rig so that we can fly a storm jib down low near the centre of effort, if and when. He provides a nicely designed solution which connects the backing plate right through to the forward bulkhead frame, the strongest point of this part of the boat. It will cost only another leg. I hope we are a millipede.

I must interrupt at this point. Women observe things that men don't and my husband's description of the owner and wife leaves too much to the imagination. Stef is just brilliant on the subject of forestays and wind vanes but I'm not sure he sees humans with the same critical attention to detail.

The Wife wears gold sandals with three inch stiletto heels. Gold toenails too. This fascinates me since most boat people either go barefoot or wear flip-flops. But this is a social visit or rather a haggling over finance visit which she leaves to her blazored husband. She is in her fifties with a perfectly even golden tan and her bronzed hair doesn't move in the wind. Her face is finished with foundation, blusher, eye-shadow, mascara, lip-liner, lipstick and anti-fouling. No, I made that last bit up. I am wearing filthy cargoes and my dusty hair is tied it up in a gypsy head scarf. The Wife looks me up and down as if I were for sale. Even cheap, she wouldn't buy me. I tell her I'm the buyer of half her boat. Not the cleaner.

She tells me her role on the boat is to entertain after a race. She wants to show me how to use the microwave and coffee-maker. Now I have a problem with this. Stef and I have given the coffee-maker to one of the yard lads and we crow-barred the microwave to make more cupboard space. I bluff about knowing how to make coffee and more or less bar her from coming on board.

'Why is she called Scrap? It's an unusual name for a boat.' I have to know this. It's been puzzling me.

'She's called Scrap because he and I are always scrapping. We scream and yell at each other. I yell from one end of the boat and he yells back from the other. Our relationship is loud!'

'I may have to change her name then because we don't yell at each other,' I say.

Well . . . only when I fail to pick up a mooring buoy or he fails to pick up the mooring when I am on the wheel. Or when he shouts Starboard! And I hear Stern! and ram the jetty.

'That would be unlucky,' She yells. 'Hey, Jock, isn't it unlucky to change a boat's name?"

Jock is yelling facts at Stef as if Stef has never seen a boat before but my husband can stand his ground. He is better than me at feigning politeness.

'Never heard that one about changing a boat's name,' he shouts back, probably to annoy her, because this myth is part of maritime folklore and familiar to most sailors.

'It's not unlucky if you don't change the first letter,' I improvise.

'Oh well, I suppose that's up to you.'

When the two of them have gone, Stef and I are a bit shell-shocked at the mismatch between Scarlet's current and future owners. We are polar opposites. Day racing versus blue water cruising. Smart and shiny versus functional and safe. Glam versus scruff (wives). Scrap versus Scarlet.

We had always hated the name Scrap and I can't remember when we settled on Scarlet. Now that we know the origin of this elegant boat's name, we are absolutely sure that she has been wrongly christened. Scarlet she is. With or without an extra T.

Bill is back and helps me identify the pumps. Every compartment of the boat has a pump, it seems: manually operated electric bilge pump, automatic bilge pump, domestic water pressure pump, deck wash pump, manual bilge pump 1, big manual bilge pump 2 (for when sinking), hand fresh water pump, hand salt water pump, diesel supply pump . . .

Meanwhile, the life raft has gone to Boston for its holidays. The shop that was definitely going to fix it on site in less than a week, a month ago, turns out not to be licensed to deal with our particular model, so it had to go to Boston, but will be with us directly, really it will.

Our visitors departed, Louis and I turn our attention to an enormous ball of unidentified rope in the bow locker. It turns out to be two, two-hundred foot lengths of heavy nylon warp, all plainly still innocent of sea water. Fifteen years in the bow locker means it won't pass for new but it should be as strong as the day it was made. We've decided, in European style, that we want full length chain on the anchor, so this nylon rope will be back-up for the second anchor, or to add length to the chain for really deep water. This may seem extravagant redundancy, but we have experience with anchors dragging and regard ground tackle as among the most important safety equipment on the boat. So Pete measures the capstan for chain size (a size heavier than the rule of thumb is my rule of thumb) and works out the price for three hundred continuous feet of galvanised high test chain. It later arrives inside a huge cardboard drum on a forklift palette, weighing several hundred pounds. I begin to worry that even with a twelve ton boat, stowing this lot in the anchor locker right up at the bow may affect our trim.

Pete maneuvers the drum on to the jetty, dumps it, and backs the forklift away. He explains that the trick is to run the chain over the jetty and into the river. The second trick is to make sure that you have a line tied to the last link, which is firmly tied to the boat. Then you haul the chain back into the boat. The line becomes the lashing onto the ring down in the anchor locker, and when the whole chain is hauled in, the anchor goes on the end fresh out the river. Pete has done this before. I like to think we would have worked it out for ourselves but I am not so sure. I have visions of us busting guts to get the half ton drum of chain over the dockside, over the rail and onto the boat, bypassing the river. Not a reassuring scenario.

Taking stock again, there are half a dozen issues still outstanding – the bimini and canvas, the satellite link, the life raft, the wind vane control lines, the inner forestay, the hot-water tank, insurance – but we can do nothing about any of them because it's the weekend.

Chapter 14

⚓

Cutting loose: one

JUNE 2005

Monday rolls round and back come the yard lads. To call them lads is to
do them an injustice; they are experienced, skilled workers, in their thirties
and forties or older, most with boats of their own. When a boatyard is run
as tightly as this one, and charges $80 an hour for its labour, the workers
have to be good. We like Fred, Bill and Pete, and always learn something
from them. They are good humoured and crack jokes at our expense until
the day we finally leave.

When we tell him that we're off for a break while we wait for stuff,
Fred suggests a little creek, just a couple of miles up river where we could
stop overnight. Bill and Pete will accompany us on this our very first outing;
Pete to give us a hand, and Bill to apply an expert ear to the gearbox under
full power. The plan is then to double back, drop Pete and Bill on the dock,
and continue up to the creek for a swim. We may even convince ourselves
that the boat is fit to leave the boatyard. After all, after fifteen years in the
yacht club, she may be agoraphobic about heading out to sea. There's even
a private mooring further up the creek which Pete and Bill happen to know
will be empty tonight. The following morning we will take her down river
to the sea, and go for a day's sailing.

We cast off. Pete steers her out. It all looks very innocent but there is
at least a knot of current under the finger piers, across the boat, and some
very expensive gin palaces to scratch. Pete has done this before. We head

out into the creek and then into the channel, past the moorings and into the main river channel. The engine and gearbox sound fine, even at full power. She's now doing what seems like a healthy 6 or 7 knots, but the log reads four. Pete isn't happy and ferrets down in the bilge to pull out the log impeller, deftly jamming his hand over the two-inch hole this extraction creates in the bottom of the boat. The log impeller doesn't seem to be weeded up. Back in it goes. I note its whereabouts. We turn around and motor back. Louis takes the helm and we drop Pete and Bill on the pier, perform a most elegant uey, and we're off to the creek. The vote to put up the sails is carried by a majority of three. Iona thinks we have enough of a challenge steering a new boat. In unknown waters. Outvoted, she hunches up against the mast and stares ahead. This girl is not happy. Her man may still choose the ocean over a safe holiday with her. Up goes the main and we unroll the enormous masthead genoa. We turn the engine off and we're gliding up river with 5 knots of wind behind us, doing a completely silent 3 knots through the water and perhaps two over the land. This is magic. We are awestruck by Scarlet's sheer size and elegance. Everything happens in a stately fashion, an impression underlined by the fact one can hardly feel that there is any wind. She is like a swan in her tutu gliding *en pointe* across the stage magically animated by some ethereal force. Before we know it, we are abeam the branch into the creek. We circle around, stow the mainsail, roll the jib, start the engine and line ourselves up with the green cans down the port side of the channel. All very unnatural for us Europeans. Now we have to rewire our reflexes for IALA Area B Buoyage: 'green right going: red right returning.'

Pete was adamant that we had to hug the right of the channel as we only have about a short foot of water to spare. We're through the narrow channel entrance and the creek widens out into a superb anchorage with about twenty boats. We cannot find the buoy we were told about but there are plenty of free ones and it doesn't look as if much traffic will come in this early in the season. About half a minute later, Scarlet is moored to a buoy, and we are all in the water – water that is as brown and cool as weak tea. Not so weak either. We each swim in our different ways from elegant breast stroke to splashy dog paddle. There are some really nice boats in here with New England classic sailing craft amongst the obligatory gin palaces, including a very elegant schooner of about forty feet. And then I realise, after a lifetime of greenly envious boat-ogling, that the blue one we are on is the most beautiful of them all.

Getting back on board is a case of kicking up into the dinghy and then climbing up from there. We have no swimming ladder yet. I sit on deck, taking it all in. The boat swings around with all the others as the tide turns. She is all-encompassingly graceful. What am I doing on this deck?

We eat. We watch the sky darken and admire the stars for a while, breathe a loud out-of-the-boatyard sigh, and turn in to sleep the sleep of the dead. In the morning, we eat breakfast, drop the mooring, and head out, hugging the port side of the channel, into the main river and back to the boatyard.

Chapter 15

Cutting loose: two

JUNE 2005

Back to the heat, the flies and the unresolved issues.

Bill persuades the new hot tank into its tight space but the engine won't restart to test the water heating. Bill goes through every wire in the stern of the boat. I'm one step behind him learning, learning, but trying to keep out of his hair. He's a very patient man and I think he's a bit bemused that an owner should take so much interest in the dirty bits. On the other hand he knows we're about to head offshore. It certainly invokes a different reaction in the yard staff than if we were just another owner moving her to another dock.

Eventually, a good six hours and several colleagues' advice later, Bill finds a connector which has popped out and disabled the fuel solenoid, apparently completely independent of the gearbox and hot-tank work. Now he can fire up the engine to give the hot-tank installation a test run. Bill's got a wonderful laser gadget that he can point at any spot and it gives him an instant surface temperature reading. This is heaven sent when you're trying to find out which is the out and which is the return from the bunch of eight pipes running through the very tight bilge space. The hot tank is declared as good as new.

Now to return to the more complicated business involving humans. The yard boss, Al, phones the broker with the bill for the tank. Steam rises from the phone. The broker phones the owner, and a couple of hours later gets back. They will graciously accept the bill for the water tank. We set up an appointment for the broker, yard owner, and myself to negotiate the final agreement of the other bills. In three days time; it can't be done sooner.

That evening we get the second installment of the bimini and dodgers. Carter-the-Canvas brings the canvas shapes he has cut from the paper templates he made last time. The bimini can be fitted to its frame in the shop, but the dodgers need a dress fitting here first before being sewn in the shop. That will take another two days.

More waiting, but look on the bright side. We have time for another escape and might even get out of the river.

This time we know the cast-off drill and make for the open sea. The river is wide, maybe a mile wide but the navigable channel is only about fifty yards wide in places and the rest is mostly one foot deep. We meander down under the road bridge which looks perilously low. Our mast is the best part of seventy feet so in the middle of the span there should be ten feet to spare, but I can only bear to peep between my fingers as we pass under it, certain that we will crundle the top five feet of mast. As we glide under, I wait for the scraping of concrete. Silence.

After the road bridge, we test the VHF by calling the railway bridge operator who says the bridge will be open in ten minutes. We chase our tail round in circles, and then we are out, through the final dog leg of dredged channel, green-to-the-right-going, past the lighthouse and into the sound. Hoist sails, check the chart, and we ghost along, heading for the gap in the rock ledges towards Long Island in a weak hazy breeze. The motor is off. We glide in a spine-tingling silence at about 3 knots across the sound. The haze is such that in half an hour we've lost all but the ghostliest whisp of the lighthouse without gaining any hint of the far shore. There are, as always, too many functions to check out, but I refuse to let it spoil the peace. The echo-sounder says that the rock ledge is where it should be, the speed through the water is just what we would guess, the compass heading agrees with the chart plotter. The GPS speed even agrees with the log, and the tables say there is no tide running. We have technology in harmony, for a change.

I wonder if there's enough breeze to test the wind vane? It hardly seems likely, but we'll give it a go. We dig out the light weather vane – a big plastic wafer – and clamp it into the top bracket. I drop the vane's hydrofoil down into the drink, adjust the bearing of the vane, and watch the control lines tighten as the hydrofoil twitches right, causing it to pendulum out to starboard. This pulls the lines. The lines turn the wheel, the boat heeds the rudder, and the pendulum drops down again, the lines loose. Even at 3 knots across the wind, it works straight out of the box. The Monitor, soon dubbed the Minotaur, following a slight speech error by the captain, is a pussycat. Just watching those beautiful, greened bronze gears working slowly back and forth, adjusting, adjusting, readjusting, is balm on nerves jangling with boatyard hassles. The big boat just keeps on gliding. In our previous boat, which was no slouch, this would have been only enough wind to keep her steerable, even by hand. But with 5 knots of wind and the wind vane steering, Scarlet is happily gliding along at 3 knots. The wind drops entirely for a minute or two but the twelve tons of boat just keeps on going, picking up speed as the breeze recovers.

By lunchtime, Long Island is just reliably differentiating from the mist. Careful attention to bearings over ten minutes or so says that the tide is gaining eastward. Through the binoculars I can see beach houses and the odd mansion.

Too soon, and with an enormous collective sigh, it is time to go back to the boatyard and the negotiations. As we head back, the sea breeze picks up. It is a magic, muted sail. In we go, past the lighthouse, into the channel, lucky this time because the bridge is up, and within an hour we are docking her at the jetty. Louis handles her beautifully. He notes that there is no pronounced paddlewheel kick from the propeller and admires her manners.

So here we are tied up to our pitch again. We fetch dinner from the deli. The sea air and a huge sense of relief have us all bunked by ten.

CHAPTER 16

⚓

Boatyard blues

JUNE 13TH 2005

This is when it should all come together. The life raft arrives from Boston and costs half the estimate, which is a nice surprise. The forestay goes in. Carter-the-Canvas arrives and fits the bimini and dodger. Wow! Stylish! We were hesitant about the choice of colour, but the pale tan, traditional on New England boats, looks stunning against Scarlet's dark blue hull and teak decks. Fifteen days late, but stunning. And they fit her like haute couture. The inner forestay came this morning and was fitted, all in twenty minutes. The missing jib has been found and delivered, as well as a storm jib which the broker has bought second hand to replace the one that wasn't. We now know that the satellite system is not going to be delivered in time, though we think we might be able to buy one, or an alternative, in Newport over the counter. We'll finish off the wind vane control lines tonight.

Outstanding is the small matter of settling up. I have been paying for each of the items that were clearly down to us as they were done. The yard owner says that the broker is arguing about who pays for the antifouling, the hot-water tank, and various other items such as stepping the mast (not re-stepping; we have already paid for that). I phone the broker who gives me his line. No-one asked for the antifouling to be done. The hot tank would never have rusted if the yard had wintered the boat properly. Bill must have broken the electrical connector which prevented the engine restarting, so they're not paying for the many hours spent sorting the problem. The broker suggests I authorised the tank work at a ridiculous price without asking him. Did we discover that the water tank was totally rusted on the same day as the survey because if it wasn't, then the escrow won't cover it and we would have had to pay? Just out of interest, I tot up how much is being charged to the escrow money and find that the damage comes to almost exactly the $10,000 set aside.

My main thought is how lucky we are that the tank bust when it did. A day later and we would have been liable for payment, and a month later and we would have lost half our water mid-Atlantic. Some things don't bear thinking about! I put down the phone and the yard owner goes through *his* case. The antifouling was done even before we ever set eyes on the boat, as part of the over wintering. He is adamant that it is down to the previous owner and agrees with me that we are not responsible for payment. And he is just as dismissive of the idea that the tank problems were bad layup or that the electrical fault is a result of some damage Bill did in fitting the tank. So he's all on our side. We set up a meeting with the broker, owner, and yard but this can't possibly happen for another four days.

We arrived on May 31st and it's now June 13th. The hurricane season is creeping up on us. We have to get to Newport to exit the US and be clear of Bermuda before late June to satisfy the insurance, and for our own self-preservation. Already there has been one hurricane down in the Caribbean, subsequently downgraded to a tropical storm, but reminder enough.

I wonder what would happen if we just sail off. I imagine that they have some way of getting the Feds to stop us through a lien on the boat – I'm getting quite nifty with US legal jargon. On the other hand, I'm absolutely happy that we've paid up on every item which we owe. The yard owner's argument with the previous owner is none of our business. If we were sold a boat that was anti-fouled the first time we ever saw it, then the paint is in the price – an inalienable part I think they say – but however right we are, these are people with lawyers. All they have to do is delay us a couple more weeks and we cannot get the boat out this year. They could easily delay for months and cost us a fortune. What's more, they know that, and they know we know that. Not a very strong wicket to bat on. My grandmother-in-law once told me, as I headed to the US as a much younger man: 'Stay out of the hands of the doctors and the lawyers and you'll have a great time!' I never found out what her experience was but I took her advice. It proved good advice. The yard owner has been very friendly and I suspect that underneath the businessman veneer his sympathies are probably with us, but he has staff to pay and his lawyers would say that possession is nine-tenths of the law. Funny how international that expression is. Finally, after a few more times around the bush, he tells me straight: You can't leave. We'll impound you! This after informing me that there is absolutely no case for our being responsible for any of the remaining bills. OK, so if we are going to do a fully justifiable runner, we must give not the slightest hint, so instead of asking him about the mechanics of impounding, I explain that my wife is not in the best of health and that another four days baking in the boatyard might kill her. Then the lawyers really would have a field day.

As a sop he offers us one of his moorings out in the river which is a whole lot cooler than being tied to the jetty. I explain that this is very kind but we desperately need more sea trial time to find any further problems before we set off into the blue. I promise we'll be back on Thursday, and finally he relents and says: 'Just so long as you are!' In the end he is a sailor first and a businessman second.

⚓

CHAPTER 17

Cutting loose: three

We motor out to the mooring for the night and plan our next sea trial – a two-day voyage over to Long Island, round Montauk Point and across the Inner Sound. For the first time, we're going to cross a bit of sea.

The voyage down river and across to Long Island is much as before, perhaps a bit more wind, but not much. The VHF weather report robot says there will be 15 knots in eastern Long Island Sound but we have no more than eight. We reach the lighthouse off Montauk point, after cruising at 5 to 6 knots on a beam reach. In the gap between the point and Long Island, the wind picks up to about 12 knots and we start to feel the power of our rig. We are heeled over 15 degrees – the little U-shaped sight-glass tells us that exactly – as we round the lighthouse at 7 knots with a swoosh and a gurgle. Going through into the Inner Sound – the sea inside Long Island's lobster-claw east end – we swap one misty expanse for another. There's no sign of the other claw which is only about five miles away. This light wind, murky visibility, smooth sea, is typical of the Sound in the summer. We had intended doing a circumnavigation of Shelter Island, but by now it is late, and the sky has greyed over, and, as usual, we are all tired. The boatyard business is utterly exhausting – the lists, the modifications to the lists, the hassles – so we opt for a sheltered looking anchorage which is right inside a landlocked lagoon on the South claw. We put in a couple of tacks to get us round the headland and lined up with the narrow entrance. She beats beautifully. She can quite comfortably make 45 degrees off the true wind, maybe even a hair better when we've learned to trim her perfectly. That's fine by me.

The entrance channel is no more than 20 yards wide with only about a foot depth to spare in places so we all concentrate furiously, Lynn at the helm, and Louis up front on rock watch while I scrabble about in the pilot book reading off the buoys. It is not terribly clear where the sand spit ends. We take a chance, throw her over to starboard, and squeak into the lagoon. The anchor goes down in ten feet of water, and we're only a couple of hundred yards from the marina for supplies. Very snug. Four other boats are already anchored; that's enough to feel as if we're where we think we are. Coming in for the night somewhere snug, even after such a trivial voyage, is always special.

The only blot is that we discover that we have no bread. This is not serious, but an excuse for a little exploration. Louis and I dinghy to the small marina, tie up and find out that the shop closed half an hour ago. It's still early season, not that it looks as if there is anything of much use to man nor beast in there anyway. Through the window we see mainly sailing apparel tending toward the brass button blazer genre. Apparently we are in the Hamptons. My Long Island geography is hazy, but even I have heard of the Hamptons which I associate with Gatsby. The mansions seen through the binoculars look congruent. Only the restaurant is open, with a menu dominated by lobster and a right hand column requiring pre-administration of a stiff whisky from the aperitifs section. The head waiter greets us surprisingly genially given that we are clad in our old jeans and sandals, and offers us half a dozen upscale bread rolls covered in rare seeds. He won't dream of payment.

Back on Scarlet, we drink cold beer out of the freezer, eat our free and fabulous bread rolls, and pass out again. The latter, by now, could be called a habit.

Next morning we set off back to boatyard purgatory. There is a moment of hubris, a slight glitch, when we run aground ever so gently on the sand bar in the middle of the main channel, and yes, it is mentioned in the pilot though it seems to have moved and is unmarked. Fortunately the tide is flooding so a quarter of an hour later we are out in the open sea, though not before a New York State Ranger launch has hailed us and asked whether we have our season's cruising license. We explain the boat is UK registered though we have not yet changed the 'NY, NY' on the stern, one of the jobs we had listed before the rather more fundamental ones took over. This is slightly delicate. Foreign yachts are supposed to have a different kind of cruising permit. I hadn't even got around to worrying about that, rather hoping that we might be allowed to make it up the coast to Newport, bowing out of the US without one. Just as I am about to launch into a rather complicated explanation, he smiles broadly and says: 'Just checking, I don't want to see it.'

I think he is amused that we ran aground on the sandbar. I'm quite happy to look an absolute idiot if it saves a night in jail. So we retrace our tracks, and by evening we're back up river and tied up on the all too familiar jetty.

The following morning there is good news on the insurance front. After numerous toings and froings with Martin in Annapolis, he's fixed us up with a policy, ironically underwritten by Lloyd's of London. They're happy as long as the yard writes a letter vouching that a professional rigger has disassembled and checked the standing rigging. Pete is a professional rigger if ever there was one, so the yard writes us a letter which is faxed to Martin. The rest of the policy is fairly standard, some gobbledegook alerts and warnings about nuclear invasions, but I note that the only directly relevant thing is that we're not covered for named storms in Bermuda after July 12th and before November 30th. So if we make it to the Canaries we're OK. And if we stay on the east coast we are OK. Insurance is the biggest single running expense of the year, but unavoidable.

Today is Wednesday and we are set up for the denouement in the four cornered ring on Thursday: broker, owner, buyer, yard.

7 a.m.
Pete and Fred and Bill, neat in Ferry Cove Boatworks t-shirts and white socks, wake us with their jokes and teasing.
'Still here? '
'Thought you were going to cross the Atlantic?'
It has been like this for a fortnight, men crawling over, inside, and around the boat while we try to live on board. Now the tension mounts as the four way negotiation over who pays for all this labour at $80 an hour

(previous owner, ourselves, broker, boatyard) reaches a nasty stalemate with much shouting down mobile phones.

10 a.m.

The thermometer outside the office registers 100 degrees in the shade; it is sticky, muggy and still. Our boat is tied to the quay and going nowhere. My husband walks between the boat and the office. The boat and the office. Our brains boil as the temperature, emotional and meteorological, mounts. We tell them that we are setting sail right now because we can't stand another day in the boatyard shouting and arguing, but they tell us we will be arrested and the boat impounded. The bill, very large, has to be settled.

5 p.m.

The hire car went back long ago, but Ed, the owner of the boatyard, very kindly hands us the keys to the yard pickup when the men go off duty so that we can go and start on provisioning and carting back drinking water. Louis has a great time with the 300 horse, air-conditioned truck. First right at the train tracks, and into the mega-mall out of town. So far we have been living off expensive sandwiches from the deli and the only six edible and affordable items supplied by a limited and exorbitant village grocery store. Americans don't buy food locally.

We buy enough food to feed several armies. I concentrate on the nourishing items in the cold aisles – milk, fruit juice, yoghurt, cheese, smoked meat – while my son assures me that I am doing this all wrong because what we need are thirty tins of soup, thirty tins of ready meals, and thirty packets of chocolate biscuits, a decision which will prove uncannily accurate and shaming for his mother. Real sailors avoid the cold aisles, he tells me with confidence. Three full trolley loads which cost several hundred dollars are ferried back to the boat in the truck. Husband and son leave me to stow the food mountain while they return to the supermarket for water. It is dark when they arrive back with fourteen two-gallon plastic containers of water. I photograph the huge jars lined up on deck under the moonlight – a surreal photo. Louis tells me that a check-out assistant inquired, straight-faced, as they were rolling the tons of water past the till:

'Paper or plastic?'

We celebrate with a very late supper of steak and raspberries. Now we are too full to sleep. Too hot to sleep. Too hot.

CHAPTER 18

⚓

Last day in the boatyard

JUNE 14TH 2005

I think the boatyard is at last tiring of their scruffy and increasingly bad-tempered British residents who lower the tone of their expensive garage facility for smartly dressed owners of polished motor boats who arrive for a little trip up river and back.

Proper sailors like us can't help laughing at the importance of cosmetics. Gangs of men, balanced on scaffolding and planks, polish and buff the motorboats. Rub rub, rub. Men in baseball caps and shades. Men with naked torsos, sweat pouring down their backs, shining up miles of paint.

Across the river opposite the boatyard, only a hundred yards away, is a posh island marina with shower-block, launderette, pool and café. A little red ferry manned by a smart Red-Shirt takes bona-fide boat owners in white socks and sandals back and forth, back and forth, all day. One minute there. About turn. One minute back. A bee buzzing through its day. At first we successfully hitch lifts despite the lack of appropriate footwear, and the Red-Shirt doffs his cap to us. But they have wised up that we are the three grotty Brits in the pounded yacht so we have to wait for the cover of night to hop on and get a shower or put a wash on. I reckon we might as well use the facilities while we are stuck here.

I put on a sun-dress, put towels and shampoo into a bag, step onto the ferry and cross. Wow! The showers! Each cubicle in a private, separate room with chintz wicker chairs and sofas, huge mirrors, boxes of tissues in matching chintz containers.

Thursday, the serious games begin. These guys have played before. The yard owner has been surreptitiously rehearsing me for this, I realise. In private, he's not fond of the owner whom, he says, he won't have back in the yard with another boat for all the tea in Boston harbour. I'm not quite sure I believe him, but I don't envy him the job of dealing with the rich. I find it hard to take against the yard owner because the yard crew have been absolutely great. They've been really supportive of this weird English family who actually live on the boat while it's being fixed and who are somewhat green when it comes to a trip across the pond. They are all sailors in their very small amount of spare time, and they seem to be behind us, regarding us with a mixture of incredulity and solicitude. It is obvious that they regard Scarlet as their flagship. Almost everything else in the yard is a gin palace and we're setting off into the big blue in the jewel in their crown. They want us, and her, to arrive in one piece, wherever. Whatever.

The bargaining begins. The mast re-stepping is ours; the anchor chain is ours. The hot tank job cost $3000. Unhappiness abounds. There is an argument about whether it was found before, during or after the survey, and whether the charge is reasonable, and whether I authorised the work without consulting the broker. Yes, no and no. I have already paid the difference between stainless and rustable; about $100. I don't see that the yard's charge to the owner is any of my business. I point out that the whole process has not been helped by the elasticity of the inventory. First there is an SSB, a storm jib and an inner forestay, but no running backs. Then there is no SSB, no storm jib. There never was an inner forestay but there are running backs. How am I supposed to get ready for a trip across the Atlantic? These aren't cosmetics; they are basic safety equipment. We have already traded the new bimini and dodger, the running backs and the forestay for the SSB. Not a bad deal for them.

12 noon.
The previous owner is insisting we pay half of a very expensive paint job on the hull which we did not ask for and knew nothing about. More

shouting into mobile phones. Faxes are sent from the boatyard office. Faxes arrive back. They have us over a barrel because while Jock refuses to pay up, we can't leave. Stef walks between boat and office. Boat and office. Office and boat. Louis and I read his face as he paces back.

It's a No.

It's still No.

It's bloody No.

The final sticking point is the antifouling which was done before we set foot in the US. The broker claims that no-one requested the hull be anti-fouled, that it was anti-fouled before, and besides I'm getting the benefit. I was quite definitely told that the hull was *newly* anti-fouled and that the owner was paying, and the broker pointed out that it was indeed newly anti-fouled when we inspected it in February. And benefit is what I expect to get when I buy something. The yard can't find a written order, but they always anti foul as part of launching and show us last year's itemised bill so there's no question of them overcharging. Satisfied that my arguments are absolutely right and completely conclusive, and remembering my grandmother-in-law's advice, I decide we'll have to pay for the anti fouling.

3.15 p.m.

It's a Yes!

It's really a Yes!

Stef carries rolled up faxes. Some deal has been struck, not entirely to our advantage, he reports, and we have clearance! We can hear the boatyard boss shouting down the phone again to Jock. Before they can catch us with some new problem, we untie the ropes.

We are off.

Dozens of forms are signed and faxed this way and that. Credit cards are flourished. The yard bestows the boatyard t-shirt on the whole crew. We say our goodbyes to Pete, Fred and Bill and the rest of the yard crew. In the process we get a recommendation for Ram Island as the best first night anchorage on the way to Newport. We pile out of the office, jump into the dinghy and motor out to the mooring. We are just hoisting the sail when the yard's inflatable roars up. We scan it for bailiffs but it's the secretary and boatman with one last form to be signed. A deep communal sigh of relief and off we go again down river.

We anchor for the night a couple of miles down river and our excitement at leaving is very much submerged beneath the tension and the mounting, unspoken recriminations as Iona gets ready to leave the boat. She drags a rucksack which is larger than herself out of the cabin and onto the deck. These two young people are deeply in love, and we are about to take one of them on a trip across the ocean. Discussion between the generations has been drowned out by the hassles and arguments over the handover of the boat. No-one has had a chance to express their feelings about the venture. Iona, with some justification, thinks we are irresponsible and crazy to set off in this state. She is not speaking to Stef or me.

In silence, they get themselves and the giant rucksack down into the dinghy and I watch as Louis pulls the starter cord, and quickly I am left with only the outlines of two people in a small boat against a darkening sky. I can just about make out that the two forms do not move. One holds the tiller. One faces forward and does not look back. Then I can only see a blur and finally nothing.

Plan B has prevailed and it is a quiet and upset Louis who returns alone, climbs aboard Scarlet, and vanishes into the privacy of his cabin.

The enormity of our leaving is blanketed in silence and sighs. Our son is not happy. This evening we are subdued when we should be deliriously excited. Stef alone, perhaps, has his mind on the journey ahead.

In the morning, no-one wakes us. There are no drills or cranes, no buzzing ferry, no anger. We up anchor and set off for Newport.

We are on our way to Newport.

Is it true?

Do we believe it?

CHAPTER 19

To Newport

JUNE 14TH 2005

In the morning, not very early, Scarlet exits the channel by the lighthouse and turns to port instead of heading out into the sound. There are rock shelves along the coast so navigation is not completely straightforward, but there are fairway buoys at intervals so neither is it particularly arduous. By maintaining a course about a mile off shore we miss the hazards. The breeze is a gorgeous, 15 knots on the beam and we plough along, all three in the cockpit, finally unwinding like a ball of rubber bands. The wind vane is doing its stuff – still a source of wonder.

At this pace it will be about four hours to Ram Island, with ETA around dusk. We watch the landmarks pass, occasionally scanning with the binoculars, marking off the anchorages. We pass several distant forests of masts which mark marinas and yachting centres. No-one is saying much, glad of the new peace. I refuse to update the mental lists. This is where I thought we would be about two weeks ago but here we are, quite a bit poorer in dollars than predicted, but let's say richer in experience. The wind holds up and we close Ram Island well before sunset, watching the shelving bottom on the echo sounder while we sail round the back of the island and drop the hook. We do not even bother the engine. Scarlet drops back onto the anchor and the chain pulls up taut. A biting anchor always cheers the skipper. Louis takes the dinghy ashore to interview the sheep, but Lynn and I just sit on the foredeck and drink in the silence.

Love the image, Stef, but we must be truthful with our readers and tell them that our son's thoughts and emotions are elsewhere, and that he has left the boat to get away from his parents. It has been a difficult time for the two young ones, closeted and cohabiting with preoccupied in-laws (I use the term loosely) on a boat tied up to a jetty in searing heart with everyone frantic and often tense and upset. I would not recommend living on a boat with anyone unless you already know them extremely well or are super-sociable. Neither of these conditions applied. Some sailors just love company. I don't. It's hellishly claustrophobic down below, and where do you go when you want a good long break from the others? I desperately need my own space and solitude. Iona too perhaps. So despite the unrelenting blue sky, she has left under a large black cloud which in turn dumps rain on Louis. He is gone a very long time.

Let's just say that it has been very hard on everyone. Stef and I tried to carry on as usual only with a ton of tasks to complete before we set sail, while tripping over two moony young lovers. The honcho at the boatyard had to ask us, red-faced, to ask them to stop kissing and groping in full view of all the lads! They spent as much time as they could away from the boat – on the beach, in the village, anywhere. The girlfriend did not want her boy crossing an ocean with his crazy parents and, we guessed, was exerting a fair amount of pressure to stop him going. Louis did his best to help us and took on some rotten jobs like folding himself into the back locker to fit the wind vane. He did not shirk but he worked under duress. He must have felt very torn.

Night falls and suddenly it's getting chilly. At first I attribute feeling cold to all the fresh air and sunburn, but it is not just that. There's a change in the air which I predict is a weak cold front. No late evening lounging on deck for us tonight. We eat supper and do our customary passing out.

Next morning Scarlet sits in a New England mist. After the 100 degree days in the boatyard this is more like the NW Scottish coast. We add more layers and head out under engine, waiting for the breeze, following the line of buoys round the islands and past the tide race which is slack just now. The wind fills in from the north east, on the nose, and a bit stronger than we've seen so far, but only about 15–20 knots. Now we're going to find out how Scarlet beats.

We take a four mile tack out, almost back to Long Island. The sea is grey, the air is grey, the wind is cold, and we're fairly pressed, under full canvas, as we make between 6 and 7 knots hard into the wind. It turns out that Scarlet is what they call a 20/20 boat. She heels 20 degrees when beating into 20 knots of wind under full sail. A real stiff cruising boat, very different from our previous plastic fantastic which would have been over on her ear by now. Although I have not yet experienced this first hand, it's not difficult to appreciate how much energy this will save on a long passage. Sail trimming is fun, but repeated reefing drains energy from a small crew on a long voyage.

However, she doesn't seem to be pointing nearly as well as she did during the other two days in the Sound. She seems blunt this morning. You feel it in your stomach as much as anything, a feeling akin to having left the hand brake on. Your eyes are doing the calculations and the distant landmarks are not moving properly. The log and the GPS are at odds again, and a bit of homework with the tide tables indicates that the tide turned against us an hour earlier than I had calculated, a full 2 knots, maybe a bit more this close to the tide race. I've insulted her. She's not blunt: we're just crossing a fast moving stream.

We turn on the VHF radio for the robot's weather forecast. She says it's currently 51 degrees Fahrenheit. Later we hear on the local radio station that this is the coldest temperature recorded in June for sixty years. Just like home! We are now tacking along the shore of the island which is steep with deep water right inshore, but staying in close cheats the tide a bit and affords a good view of the island and the lighthouse on the end of the long sand spit, with a buoy a good mile off the end. The cross current flowing over the spit lets us sneak past the buoy without tacking.

We've been beating for nearly six hours and we're done in. We're all a bit queasy in the cold. The Newport nightlife isn't going to be troubled by us tonight. I promised myself Newport for my birthday but it's going to be Judith's Refuge instead. Not that I take much notice of promises about sailing destinations, least of all ones made by me. Or birthdays. Judith's Refuge has a very long sea wall, maybe a couple of miles long, surrounding a large acreage of mostly shallow water, with some buildings on shore. We christen it Milton-Keynes-on-Sea. Cosy it isn't but it'll do nicely for weary mariners. We have trouble picking a spot since it all looks exactly the same.

Despite the intense cold, Louis dinghies off towards the flatlands to phone his beloved, giving a whole new meaning to cold calling. Lynn worries that he is going to make himself ill by disappearing nightly into the freezing unknown and not returning for hours. We set about getting something warm for supper and feel a bit anticlimactic in this indifferent setting.

Stef's birthday. A bottle of hooch, a book and a t-shirt . . . but hang on, the temperature has dropped 30 degrees (I'm not kidding) and a gusty wind is dead against us. This isn't the weather for swims and celebrations. In full heavy weather gear, hardly believing that we have just left the dripping heat of the boatyard, we head out for Newport, tacking all the way. As the wind gets up and the sea becomes choppy, all hell lets loose below. We were not prepared for this, I say by way of excuse, as biscuits, bedding, and books hit the floor and begin their slithering dance. Louis crawls underneath the dining table to tie up the sliding water containers with yards of rope and for the second time in his life is seasick. Don't even ask about the first time because it involves brie sandwiches on a rocky ride. I know. Everything should have been secured before we set off. Louis collapses on his bunk, still in heavy weather gear, for a couple of hours. Stef remains stoic at the helm but we seem to be going slowly backwards and after several hours of this, we admit defeat and head for Port Judith. Imagine Milton Keynes on sea and you have a rough visual image, except it's shrouded in thick, freezing fog and we can't see a damn thing.

About 4.30 p.m. Louis wakes, eats two slices of stale bread and peanut butter and is sick again. I doze through the crashing and banging as all the cupboards empty their contents onto the cabin floor. I thought these catches were supposed to be good quality and keep the doors shut. Put it on the list of things to do which, only one day into our voyage, already fills a large sheet of paper. I wake again to cook bacon which we eat between slices of cardboard bread with tomato sauce, washed down with Becks. Then a treat – one mango between three of us. I must get better at this catering lark before we hit the Atlantic.

We anchor in the bay and stare at the long curve of ugly flat beach. Absolutely nothing here except a string of Wimpey holiday houses and grey sand. Despite feeling queasy, Louis does a 'because the lady loves

Milk Tray' act, rowing ashore to find a street in which there might be a pay-phone from which to call his girlfriend. We start worrying long before he returns. Has he drowned? Has he been mugged? Has he been arrested for wandering around Point Judith alone in the dead of night? You have to understand that in America, if you walk anywhere, people think you are deranged.

While the white knight charges off in the dinghy, I start dragging bedding around because, out of the goodness of my maternal heart, I am giving him my lovely hideaway bunk in the front cabin and taking the settee in the saloon for myself. I have got the sleeping arrangements all wrong, putting Louis in the saloon. A lad in his twenties needs a bit of privacy away from his parents, and I underestimated my level of tolerance for mess. I cannot step over his pile of dumped towels/clothes/CDs and chocolate Oreos every time I pass through the main cabin, and we haven't hit rough weather yet. He can put his squalor where it won't trip me.

Stef and I start on my new bed. In theory, the curved sofa converts to a spacious double bed when you lower the heavy dining table, which is fitted tight around the mast, into the jigsaw space between the ends of the settee. I have been looking forward to this. But when Fred and Peter removed the mast for the second time and refitted it, something must have shifted because now, when we slide the table down, it does not quite fit into the space. It's several inches too long. The result is a bed with a large plinth in the middle. We consider a few options:

- push the base of the mast forwards two inches so the table can drop nicely into place. Ha ha.
- take out the chocks which hold the mast in place. And risk losing the rigging?
- chop two inches off two sides of the table. I am all for this as the simplest option but the Skipper rules it out.

I'll manage, I say. We add the cushion to the table-plinth and I curl myself in a C shape on the settee on my right side with my left hip, left leg, left shoulder and left arm raised five inches above the rest of me. I can't sleep like this because I am not Nadia Comaneci. I sleep in twenty minute drifts, dreaming about beds made of concrete and Russian gymnasts. In the morning I wonder where to put the big table-shaped cushion. Every morning I wonder where to put the big cushion. Every morning I long for a bed without a plinth in the middle.

Newport, we grow nearer to thee! Finally we thaw out with a shot of Highland Park, a perfectly judged birthday present from the crew!

CHAPTER 20

The Dinky Docks

16TH JUNE 2005

Icy fog. In June!

We find the coastal weather station where a robot with a lisp says, 'a shance – of showers' over and over and over in a singsong voice until a real person says it's not been this cold in Long Island Sound in June since 1916. I can believe it.

My son is officially appointed Navigator which, he assures me, is superior to First Mate (me), and hunkers down at the chart plotter. In days and weeks to come, I will bless my son many times over for taking this role very seriously.

We motor-sail towards Newport with them outside in full heavy weather gear and me down below clearing up the explosion of stuff from yesterday. I fold towels, t-shirts, bedding. This is our first long voyage with our son on board – at least since he was small – and whereas usually Stef and I make a good pair, amicably and intuitively sharing chores above and below deck, with two men aboard I seem to have become galley slave and folder. Men don't fold things; they scrunch them up and shove them in a locker/ on a shelf/on deck/wherever.

'We don't have time to make the boat pretty,' my son informs me when I complain just a tiny weeny bit. 'We're busy doing important things like fishing.'

Oh no, he has his fishing gear out. Two lines trail out of the back.

Please don't let him catch anything. I pray to Neptune or whoever is in charge of these things, and he hears me.

We are running down the last ten miles towards Newport. We can see the cliffs either side of the two inlets, the lighthouse, the fairway buoys. So this is the temple of yachting. Many of the best sailing minds have seen this view of the entrance. We sail right up the channel, tidying up the boat as we go, and round the point.

What's left to do? We've been so engaged in hand to hand combat with the basic equipping in the boatyard that the actual voyage preparations have been on hold. The most important hole in our preparations is the lack of communications. Then there's a bunch of spare chandlery to buy – tools, shackles, emergency spares, outboard lock, waterproofs for Lynn, boots for all of us, flares – as well as a huge amount of laundry, shopping, and more shopping to do. After all of that, we must exit the US immigration service and customs, and then fill up with diesel and water. We reckon today and tomorrow should do it. So we hope to leave the day after tomorrow, weather permitting. No time to spare!

We pile into the dinghy. Newport harbour is like a collection of the last hundred years' boat show highlights. You get a crick in the neck dinghying across it, rubber necking all the gleaming mahogany. We tie up at the dinghy dock, vanish a sandwich at the first eating place on the front, and we're off and running. We soon find out that the big chandlers are on the ring road out of town. There are plenty of yacht electronics businesses in the yellow pages but none of them stock much of anything. They just install to order. It looks like West Marine on the outskirts of Newport is our only hope for communications.

Because we are hungry, we go ashore and plonk ourselves down in the first café we come to on the main drag. One mega sandwich for Louis and a polystyrene tub of clam chowder for each of us. Opposite is a chandlery but it's a touristy one – tea towels and key rings and table mats all decorated with a little navy blue compass or a silver anchor. Pictures of boats. And very expensive clothing. But in the bargain corner they have one pair of short calamine-pink wellies in my size.

First we wander into the little chandlers right on the front which seems to have survived by selling a mixture of useful stuff and tourist fodder and Lynn homes in on a pair of ankle high, violently pink wellies. She's very chuffed. We order an outboard lock for tomorrow, and find the shackles we need. Louis ferries the first round of acquisitions back to the boat. By this time there is a fairly stiff 20 knot breeze blowing across the harbour – a front clearing out the air – which makes dinghying a bit tricky and wet.

Back on foot, we pass the Newport Boatbuilding School with some of its completed restoration projects. Louis and I built an eighteen foot wooden lugger in the garage and driveway; now we experience yearnings to sign on and find out how to do it properly.

We ask directions to West Marine. Several times in several places. What is it with Americans? They don't know anything about where they live because they drive everywhere. After much random walking we end up down in the docks in a little office which has nothing to do with West Marine which is, we are told, several miles out of town in the mall, of course, but a helpful man calls us a taxi and tells us to go back to the main drag and wait. We wait. We sit on the pavement – sorry, sidewalk – where people step over us like we're rubbish. We wait twenty minutes. Thirty minutes. Finally we get our ride out of town and arrive at an airport-sized mall with a supermarket and West Marine. Why isn't West Marine in the town where there are a thousand sailors parked in the bay needing stuff? Why must we drive for twenty minutes to buy an electrical connection which will enable us to get weather faxes from our world band radio?

At West Marine we find out that they have never heard of the satellite system we want. All they have is a dongle that would make the laptop plus the Sony world band radio into a weather fax. If it works, this is what we need, and economical. Email was always a luxury. The EPIRB is for summoning help, and the Sony should provide weather forecasts. But weather faxes would be extremely useful. It's very much easier to read a picture than create one from a verbal forecast, especially since the deep ocean forecasts are much less detailed. We also find some snug looking frog mens' feet which are much more practical than wellies with their good grip and tight fit on the ankles; they should keep the waves out. We choose flares – pistol version – and pick up other bits and pieces.

I start shopping in the hundred-aisle, aircraft-hangar of a supermart, feeling dizzy and queasy after all the rushing around in the heat. The men join me, and we shop and shop and shop.

I am aware of the tension here between me and my son. Louis questions my ability to stock up on enough solid protein (a whale or two and whole pig carcasses) to get us across the ocean, and, rightly as it turns out, tells me not to bother with anything from the cold sections. He says scathingly: Ask any proper sailor and they'll tell you not to bother with the cold stuff. I ignore him and pile in the butter, cheeses, cold meats, patés, yoghurts, tortillas, flat breads. I put 10 packets of super-large tortillas into the trolley. Yes, Louis. I hear you.

Lynn seems to be on top of the provisioning but Louis is keeping an eagle eye on her to make sure that his portion sizes are multiplied by eight. He throws ten of everything he fancies including an obscene quantity of Oreo chocolate biscuits on top of her sensible, maternal choices. He glares at her each time she raises a questioning eyebrow.

Later we stand outside and hail a taxi. The driver doesn't blanch at our three trolleys of food – American size trolleys. We manage to fit all fifty or so carrier bags into the boot. Off we go, the driver talking non-stop in a husky, Rhode Island accent that to my untutored ear sounds very New York; Boston is Borston and the dinghy dock is the dinky dock. He tells us he was born seventy-one years ago in Newport and used to sell stuff to real ships before all this newfangled development brought in the riff raff in plastic boats. He was the water-taxi, the ice seller, the guy with moorings in the bay. He shrugs at this moment, pauses for dramatic effect, looks in his mirror to make sure I, in the back, am listening, then tells us he sold up at exactly the wrong moment.

'Y'know, I could have been a millionaire with my moorings?'

'Y'know, I could have bought the whole of the naval docks for $250,000?'

'Y'know, a mate of mine made a million bucks selling hot-dogs on the pier?'

He doesn't draw breath.

At the dinky docks we unload, and a passing yachtie remarks, 'That should last you a day or so.'

We ferry supplies back and forth, leaving one person standing watch over the carrier bags. You know the riddle about three men and a ferry and thirty bags of shopping. The effort of negotiating a vast, unknown supermarket with thirty choices of everything has left me quite shaky. It's dark by the time we finish and we are whacked. Yet Louis speeds off in the dinghy to find a phone to talk to his beloved.

It worries us that Louis is motoring round the harbour at night on his own, even before we've had a chance to familiarise ourselves with the quirks of the outboard, but Stef checked that he has the oars with him before he set off.

What we are about to embark on is much more than a trip round Newport harbour, but the statistics show that most people drown by falling out of a dinghy within a hundred yards of shore.

CHAPTER 21

The last day on land?

17TH JUNE 2005
The wind is perfect so we are going to try to get everything done so that we can leave today, before evening. LEAVE in capital letters. LEAVE which means begin our ocean crossing. So far these words do not have much reality for any of us. They will.

Our last day on land is a marathon, even by recent standards. I put two tons of washing into a machine at the launderette which is a mile from the dinky dock while Louis and Lynn depart in search of an internet café and some hardware to allow us to get satellite weather forecasts. From the launderette I go up the hill and across town to Radio Shack where I buy a spare memory card for Louis's camera because the connection to the laptop isn't working, and we want to be able to take more than twenty pictures of our ocean journey. Then I set off for the internet café where we have agreed to meet up. I find it straight away, only to find that Lynn and Louis are not there.

We decide to split, and since Stef is the only one strong enough to carry the washing, much of it soaked with sea water from leaks on the way to Newport, he volunteers to play Hunt the Launderette while Louis and I search for Josies which, we are told, is the only internet café in Newport. The only one? Really? Louis needs to do something with Stef's laptop. Stef will meet us there.

We walk.

And walk.

By 11 a.m. it is sultry-hot. Louis drips as he carries Stef's ancient, heavy laptop all over Newport, and I drip walking beside him. I am on edge because I can see how ill he feels but when you have been ill most of your life, there comes a point when you give up discussing it. That was about ten years ago.

When we finally find the internet café, the waitress tells us we cannot plug in our own laptop; we can only use their computers. What! We need to go to a different internet café. The waitress isn't sure where it is but gestures further along the street. What I didn't know then is that when Americans gesture vaguely along a street, it means they don't know. On we go, several more blocks and road junctions, until the high street becomes a series of small, sporadic shops and scruffy cafés, and then turns into a residential district. Why don't these Americans know their own towns? They run in very small tracks, we conclude. In a two-internet-café town, you would think the waitress in the first would know where the second one is.

'If I'd plugged it in, she'd never have noticed,' Louis says. 'She doesn't even know if there is another internet café or not.'

'Stef will be on his way to Josies and not find us.'

'I don't believe there is another internet café.'

We walk further, passing a man who tells us the internet café is indeed somewhere on this very street. Further on, he says, waving vaguely into the far distance. Another urbanite who doesn't know. Further on are traffic lights and a major highway. He must have meant further back. He must have meant Josies. We turn back and head for Josies again, and after another hour of tramping the hot, dusty streets, we spot Stef in the distance standing outside the internet café, looking left then right then left. He is tetchy because of the heat and because of the washing which is in several washing machines on the other side of Newport and because no-one has found out how to emigrate.

The internet café is cool and metallic with glass chess sets and wonderful cakes. Since somehow it is already 2.30 p.m., we decide to stay there and eat our last supper. I order warm glazed pear and caramelised pecan salad. Then molten chocolate cake and ice-cream. Louis drinks several double espressos because he is feeling bloody awful and his brain is anaesthetised, but they don't help.

I go outside to find a pay-phone and dial a magic number for emigration. What is my husband making such a song and dance about? I am told that we can leave. Just like that? Yes. No need to go to the emigration control office? No. No forms to hand in? No. I return triumphant.

'We can go,' I say.

'No papers to sign?' Stef asks.

'No. We just go. We post our immigration papers to their office in Providence.'

'Post?'

'I said, Post!'

We are all tetchy.

While Lynn eats hot, volcanic chocolate pudding and Louis tried to jump-start his dead body systems with espressos, I phone the US Imigration Service from a pay phone in the middle of a deserted building site outside the café – rather surreal. It turns out that they are not interested. Incredibly, this particular guy hasn't ever faced the problem of a boat leaving Newport. Do I believe this? After consultations he says to put the green tickets currently stapled in our passports into an envelope and post them, and be gone. To begin with I wonder whether he's in Texas or perhaps Bombay, but the address he gives is in Providence, just up the road. However, I'm not arguing (for a change). If they don't record our leaving, then we'll be down as illegal immigrants, but at present we're focused on the problem of getting out.

One problem solved, one laptop problem unsolved, and one bag of washing half-solved.

Now this is weird. I know we were exhausted. I know we are overwrought – about to cross an ocean for the first time. But we each remember phoning US Immigration from the building site outside the internet café. Duh!

We split again. Louis is ashen, obviously feeling desperately ill, so he and I return to the dinky dock to sit and broil a bit more while Stef goes off to collect the washing, buy loads of fruit, and find Radio Shack to buy more memory for Louis's digital camera. And fuses, 12 volt, 3 amp, because Louis has blown a fuse on the 250DC inverter and we have no means of producing European voltage on the boat. I hope you are keeping up. I'm not. I wish we could buy new fuses for all the ones he has blown in his ME shattered body.

Stef fails to find Radio Shack.

The day is almost gone.

We are all very weary.

WE ARE NOT READY TO LEAVE.

I walk back to the launderette to pick up the clothes and buy some beer, and we're off back to the boat. What we ain't found, we don't got, as they say somewhere around here.

We spend another night in Newport.

Despite feeling ghastly, Louis goes ashore again to phone, returning at nearly midnight. I keep my mouth shut although what I want to say is: 'Dearest child, why exert all that energy trailing around town and talking on the phone for hours and then zooming about in a dinghy on black water in the dead of night when you should be in bed?' I know, I know. He is finding it hard to cut himself adrift from his girlfriend as he sets off across the Atlantic. She is scared for him, scared of boats, scared of water, and he regrets agreeing to come. He would probably rather catch a plane home.

My poor son. This should be an adventure and already it is an ordeal because you are not fit. Your parents are causing you GBH. I feel ashamed.

And it's not our last day on land.

CHAPTER 22

⚓

Last day on land

18TH JUNE 2005

I log on, make some last minute checks on email, and then get up a NOAA weather forecast. The relevant offshore areas Cape Fear and Hudson Sea Canyon read: North 15-20 knots for the next three days, then backing NW. Getting off the north east US coast was always going to be the trickiest part of our journey. It's a question of timing our exit relative to the big depressions that clear off the land onto the Atlantic at fairly regular intervals, about once a week. North is not great because the Gulf Stream runs north and so a north wind generates a wind-against-current situation with some nasty steep seas. If a north wind were to shift north east, then it would effectively be a headwind in those conditions. If it backs NW, as forecast, then that should be fine. I figure that 20 knots is not huge, and perhaps we can afford to be pushed a little south at the beginning. After all, lots of crews go by way of Bermuda voluntarily. Needless to say, both I and the crew are eager to be off, and clear of the hurricane season. And there's the small matter of the day job to get back to. Waiting for a fairer wind with more west in it might take a week. The breeze in the bay the day before yesterday was probably the sign of the exact right moment to go, but we still needed two days of preparations before we were ready. Without much agonising, we decide to give it a go anyway. Just a few more errands first.

Back in the un-serious chandlers which specialises in nautically-themed knick-knacks, I buy some expensive waterproof trousers as an insurance policy, and ask the shop owner if there is a shop nearby where I can buy last-minute fresh stuff like eggs that haven't been in cold storage. And bread. And matches. We still don't have matches.

'You're English! You can walk!' the chandler owner says, and sends us off on a mile shlep uphill to another goddam shopping mall.

'I said we only wanted eggs and matches,' I complain.

'In America, this is where you buy eggs and matches. You expect a corner shop or what?'

'Yes,' I sulk. 'Why not?'

'But look!' He shouts. 'There's Radio Shack!'

And a wholefood shop where we buy four dozen un-refrigerated eggs like you're supposed to for keeping on a boat, and some Green & Black chocolate. And matches. I send apologies downhill to the woman in the chandlers.

Then we stand in Radio Shack for about three hours. Well, I stand and Stef talks to the guy. This is the most boring shop in the world; I am not remotely interested in technology. Out of sheer boredom I buy a child's walkie talkie set so that I can hear at the helm whether Stef, in the bows, is shouting port or starboard. Stef buys a memory chip for Louis's camera.

Back on the boat. The memory is the wrong kind of memory. The chip itself works but Louis still can't download photos on to the laptop. The walkie-talkie doesn't work because we don't have the right batteries. So: Louis has exactly 40 photos on his digital camera for an entire cross-Atlantic trip. He deletes old photos to make a bit more space. Neither method of getting photos from the camera to the laptop works because of some freaky behaviour unique to our laptop.

OK. Forget the technology for now. Again it is mid-afternoon and we are not spending another damn night in Newport.

Shall we go?

Yes

Yes

Yes

That's three votes for leaving.

We motor to the fuel pier on Goat Island where Louis parks our boat perfectly alongside the quay. The water tanks are filled. The fuel tank is filled. Louis demands a last hamburger like a man on death row. I jump ashore but there is no shop or takeaway, only an expensive eat-in restaurant. My last memory of leaving Newport is of tears pouring down my cheeks as I fry onions and mince so that Louis can have the 'with everything' hamburger he is longing for. I miss the departure from the fuel pier. When I emerge from the galley, mission accomplished, we are heading out of Newport. The wind has gone. We motor, for once without complaint from the Skipper, because we need to charge the batteries so that we can get the fridge cold.

It's rather late in the afternoon when we pull up at the diesel pier, fill up fuel and water, donate the kiddies' lifejackets which we can't stow, and point Scarlet out to sea. The folk at the fuel dock must be used to being the last contact with land for departing seafarers but for seafarers like us, for whom this is the first time, it is with fast-beating hearts and an overwhelming sense of unreality that we cast off. There should be some way of marking the start of the passage. Where are the flares? The good wishes? The clink of champagne glasses?

Of course we are all apprehensive but it is such a relief to stop shopping that, at this point, the fact that we are setting off to cross the Atlantic hardly figures. The preparations, the intricate planning and the angst have been relentless since we landed at the airport twenty days ago, and before that, for months, we had ploughed through an ever-extending list of jobs. The hardest part of the whole process has been to keep thinking strategically while drowning in detail. We're pleased with ourselves that we're here at all.

When the rooster crows at the break of dawn
Look out your window and I'll be gone . . .
Next stop the Canaries!

This should feel momentous but motoring out of Newport is just like motoring out of any other place en route to the next and it is impossible to crank up an appropriate emotional response. I want a banner trailing from the boat, like newlyweds leaving for their honeymoon, saying: First Time Across The Pond.

PART TWO

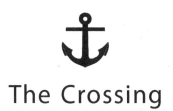

The Crossing

CHAPTER 23

Into the blue

18TH JUNE 2005

I'm getting in the fenders, and trying to seal off the hawse pipe where the anchor chain exits the chain locker. The hole is an awkward shape and hard to plug. I have unshackled the anchor from its chain and stowed it below, under the focs'le berth. We won't be needing it for a while.

The wind is light, about 4 knots SW. There is a flurry of tiny racing dinghies with junior helmsmen whizzing about the channel as we leave Newport for the ocean. We are happy to motor for a while to charge the batteries and soon we are passing the last of the buoys. The twelve meter ex-neighbour swishes past us on its way back into harbour. Soon we are out of sight of land and a couple of hours out, the batteries are full. I turn the engine off and we're back to our old gliding habits. At least there's some sun now, hazy but quite warm.

Louis decides on a bit of fishing. On the advice he got from the local tackle shop, he bought some lures especially for fishing off a sailing boat. He was also told that once we're past the Gulf Stream, there's zilch fish until the Azores. Lynn is not happy about fishing. Several moral philosophy debates ensue about murderous fishermen and hypocritical fish eaters, which I manage to stay out of on the assumption that he won't catch anything. Soon two lines are trailing out astern.

More usefully, we have a debate about watch keeping and decide that Louis will do evenings, Lynn will do nine to midnight, and I will take the graveyard shift from midnight until someone can be dragged out of their bunk. During the day we'll be more flexible, but make sure that someone is designated. The textbooks advise rotating shifts so that each crew member's watch times change from day to day, but that seems a recipe for no sleep at all. I'm much more adaptable about my sleeping than the other two who need their sleep since being ill, and so I think I can handle the early hours, but only if there is a fixed rhythm to it.

I'm at the helm – at least I'm supervising the minotaur – while Lynn gets some rest before her night shift and Louis is sitting up front. I've got the boat trimmed and we glide along at 3 knots in barely more wind. I am faffing with the trim as if we were competing in a three mile race, still a bit manic about the sail being just right to keep the boat moving. Must get used to having the engine off, I tell myself! Just how long is it to the Azores at 3 knots? Lots of mental arithmetic. I lean over and put a finger on the starboard fishing line. It's vibrating. Having not felt it before, I'm not very sure. A childhood of fishing has taught me the axiom that you never catch anything in the first week. The line has been out about an hour and I don't want to disturb Louis, so I haul it in a bit, and soon I'm sure that it is a fish.

'Louis, there's a fush!'

Family joke. Mock Scots, like mulk for milk and jum for gym. Lun for Lynn. He comes scrambling back, and I hand him the line while I go digging in the cockpit locker for the kids' fishing net to help it aboard. The fish is wound in and looks a healthy size. I lean over and net it while Louis hauls in. We have three pounds of beautiful bluefish (I think) flapping on the deck. I dispatch it with a winch handle. Blood everywhere and a certain amount of thrashing, but I'm fairly sure it's well out of it. I was better at this when I was twelve, less conscious of my own mortality or something. Louis is like the Cheshire Cat. Lynn is screaming moderately from somewhere in the cockpit. This subsides. Then Louis notices that the other line is out at 45 degrees to the wake. And its not the minotaur that has done a sneaky left turn. He grabs the line and winds in and soon another three pound bluefish is netted and banging about on deck. Louis winch-handles it. More blood. More screams, higher pitched, from the cockpit. Out with the kitchen knife and we haul a bucket full of sea water up. The nice teak decks are covered in gore, as are we. Fillets are stacked in a bowl. Lynn expires.

It is our first evening out on the ocean. I sit in the cockpit, my face in the wind and sun, trying to get a grip on reality. Louis has fixed two fishing lines which trail from our bows, but I am relaxed about this because, based on past experiences, his chances of catching anything are slim.

'Wow! Got a fish. Got a big fish!'

Louis is treading on me to get to the stern and is pulling in the line. I bury my head so that I can't watch. I hate this.

'You're a hypocrite!' He says, as he reels in the line. 'You go to Tesco and buy a piece of fish and eat it without complaining.'

'I'm a hypocrite,' I agree. 'I prefer not to recognise what I eat as fish.'

'Go away!' he says, 'if you're going to pull faces.'

Now there is a fish on the other line as well. Two fish. I stare resolutely out to sea, over the stern, while dull clubbing noises reach my blocked ears. Louis uses one of the winch handles to belt the life out of two large Bluefish. With the fish finally dispatched, he uses his penknife to turn the creatures into fish fillets. Blood everywhere. The stink of fishy death.

'Oh my god!' I say over and over.

'Shut up!' They both shout back.

The other two cook three pounds of fish with boiled potatoes and green beans. They swoon over the freshness of their protein and congratulations flow from father to son. I eat the potatoes and green beans.

Since it happens to be dinner time, fish supper is set to fry. Lynn has un-volunteered for cooking duty. This is our first mutiny after only six hours afloat and not in international waters. But Louis's catch of two magnificent fish has become a bountiful meal. He and I manage almost all the first one. The rewards of the hunter are to be seen in his primitive grin.

CHAPTER 24

First night's watch

Soon after leaving Newport, we cross the shipping lanes with barely any traffic in sight. We're headed out east, crossing well south of Nantucket and its shoals. The waters are deep but are a ship's graveyard. The wrecks are mostly a long way below our keel so the only stationary thing to hit out here is ODAS 44008 Fl. (4) Y 20s, a meteorological buoy. Ninety degrees magnetic will give it a good wide birth. We won't even see it. That's about it for the night. The wind has picked up a certain amount now, about 10 knots from the north, and we're making good progress easterly, nearly 6 knots, busy digesting dinner, watching the hazy sun set.

It's getting a bit chilly.

Lynn comes on watch, Louis and I go down to get some sleep. Louis has swapped shifts with Lynn tonight, something to do with the fish I suspect. I am soon fast asleep in the starboard single bunk in the saloon, leaving the captain's double in the rear cabin free so that navigation can go on unhindered.

8 p.m.

My first watch.

The boat is going like a train. We have 15-20 knots of wind which has now shifted to the NE so we're sailing into choppy waves. This is my first real watch and I take it very seriously. I sit in the cockpit feeling like a bit of an idiot and start the visual merry-go-round. I stare at the black sea. I look up at the sails, look at the telltales, look at the compass, look at the wind speed and knots, check the wind vane, scan the horizon for tankers bearing down on us. Start again. I stare at the sea . . . When I look at the clock, and I'm trying very hard not to look at the clock, I see that five minutes have passed. For a change, I sit down below at the nav table and stare at the little, green, luminous boat on the computer screen. This is not fun. What do others do for four hours in the dead of night with nothing but the black sea to amuse them?

By midnight when I wake Louis, a thick, icy-cold fog has blanketed Scarlet. We turn on the masthead strobe light. It's that bad. The bilge pump starts running which means there is water coming in down there. Stef unblocks the filter but it is still running. We are shipping water. No-one sleeps.

When Louis finally climbs into his bunk in the early hours he discovers that sea water is pouring through the two dorade vents, as well as down the hawse pipe into the chain locker. By two in the morning we are wading in several inches of water which slops uphill and downhill across the cabin floors.

Scarlet picks up speed and ploughs on through heavier and heavier seas in the cold fog.

The next thing I am aware of is being woken by Louis at about 2 a.m. He leaves me for a few minutes to surface. I'm dimly aware of a flashing light. I stumble into my warm clothes and waterproofs, frogmen's feet to boot, and out into the cockpit. The flashing is our masthead strobe. We had it fitted with the new tricolour when the mast was unstepped. I remember from my yacht master course that at some stage somewhere they were illegal, but Pete seemed to think they are standard, and I'm certainly not arguing now. I am prepared to commit quite a few minor crimes if they improve our chances of being seen. But why is the strobe on? My sleepy brain eventually asks the pertinent question. I peer into the pitch black and realise that it's also pitch fog, Labrador current fog. It's absolutely freezing cold. Louis is done in. He's been down at the navigator's table staring at the radar which he has heroically managed to get going. We exchange acknowledgements and briefings before he heads for his bunk to warm up.

It's the start of a miserable night. The fog is absolutely penetrating and it can't be much above freezing, at least that's what it feels like. It's probably about 40 degrees Fahrenheit. The wind has picked up to about 15 knots and we're zipping along. I don't have all that much experience of fog. In the Med, in the summer, our course never ran into more than a bit of light haze. In England, Lynn and I experienced a bit of thin fog around Anglesey a few times, but in the UK when we have fog, it's usually windless fog in the middle of a high. This fog is the result of a damp wind blowing across the Labrador current – a large body of sea water with the last Arctic ice-lumps melting only a few degrees north of here. It doesn't take long to decide that this kind of fog is no fun. Maybe we should slow down, if we can? On the other hand, we do have radar, and we should be able to detect anything before it gets within three or four miles of us. The quicker we get across the Labrador current and into the Gulf Stream, the quicker we'll thaw out. We're already reefed down a notch in deference, with the genoa more than half rolled up, so I may be kidding myself that we have any options for slowing down. I'm not sure how much speed we would cut by putting another reef in the mainsail.

The best option seems to be to stare at the radar down below at the nav table where it's a whole lot warmer. There's certainly no hope of seeing anything from deck. I wedge myself across the end of the captain's double bunk, across from the radar which is on the hull side of the navigator's desk. I'm about eight feet from the screen but I reckon I can see it well enough. I spend quite a while fiddling with the functions, trying to get everything adjusted, but it's tricky. There's bugger all out here for picking up a signal. When we tested it in the boatyard, it showed us the tin shed so if there are any sheds out here coming after us, we'll see them.

It's not too cold down in the cabin, but not exactly toasty either. The screen is completely mesmerical. I develop a routine for keeping myself awake, a round of functions. Check the boat speed and heading on the chart plotter. The wind speed I can't see because the dial is in the cockpit, but I'd soon feel if there was a change. Then check the radar adjustments: gain, clutter, range, and on and on. 'Check' is not the right word. 'Twiddle' is more accurate, but twiddling means that it might approximate to correct at some point and show me the oil tanker that is bearing down on us. In fact the main worry is a fishing boat. Any oil tankers are well lost from their lanes if they run us down here. With such encouraging thoughts I keep myself occupied.

Every half hour or so I get up and move about and stick my head out to stare at the pitch black fog. I remember Michael Frayne's magical send up of Wittgenstein in the fog, wringing his hands about whether he would be able to see the fog for the fog if the fog were really there. But if he could not see it, the only reason could be fog, in which case it was there. Paradox occupies my numb mind for at least a couple of minutes. The monologue of rubbish continues in similar but even less interesting vein as the only possible way to stay awake. Four o'clock arrives, the witching hour when the blood is coldest and the mind-body problem at its worst. Keeping them together that is. The little green screen is etched on the back of my eyeballs. The sweep sweeps around, and then it does it again, and then . . . no suspense there. Plenty of suspense in our general situation but it is best not to think about that. Will we hit the oncoming fishing boat? Statistics are not very reassuring. No, try again! The statistics are good, but they don't reassure somehow when you are staring into the fog, barely able to see the mast fifteen feet in front of you. They're bound to see the strobe aren't they? Their radar should pick up our radar transmissions. The top of the mast may be sticking out of a thin blanket of fog. There are stories of old sailing ships sending people aloft to peer over the blanket but this isn't a thin blanket of fog, it's a double duvet.

Dear reader, you must understand that when my brain gives you a sample of its contents on that first foggy night at sea, it feels some obligation to be mildly interesting or informative. But when, on that night, it gave me its sample thoughts, it felt no obligation whatsoever to entertain. It was all radar sweep after radar sweep. Rubbish, rubbish, more rubbish. I longed for a period of quiet meditation when nothing went through my mind, but I would be straight asleep. Rubbish is the only way to stay awake.

I wake up and it's about six o'clock. Perhaps I just dropped off for a few minutes. Perhaps! Shameful! The routine starts up again. Sweep. Sweep. Rubbish. Rubbish. About seven, the fog starts to get lighter. That's brighter, not thinner. Now you can really see that the fog's there. Eventually, I can't take any more and I go and wake Lynn. I can't even remember whether I ate anything or not. Maybe I did. I just remember falling into my bunk.

It seems ominous to be so exhausted just one night out. It's the cold and the anxious fog that's done it.

I wake up perhaps four hours later. Louis and Lynn are both up. The motion is a good deal rougher. We're ploughing along and the sea is getting up. Our course is now well south of east with the wind round to north east. The nor'easter we were hoping would not happen is now blowing 18–20 knots. The crew is not happy. They're wet. Scarlet is taking water into the fo'c'sle. Louis goes out on deck, runs crouched and bent to the front with two plastic bags, and heroically sticks them over the dorade funnels as if suffocating a pair of glue sniffers. The water has been getting down the dorades and into the cupboard where we keep all the bedding and towels – a great place to spring a leak. Why are they leaking? The funnels are swiveled round backwards to avoid the oncoming spray, and anyway they should be able to swallow plenty of spray and let it drain out on deck. These are supposed to be the heaviest duty ventilation you can get. The drains from the dorade boxes to the deck look inadequate to me, but now is no time for a full analysis. Leave that for the post mortem, but not literally I hope.

We are all not just wet but green. On one particularly thorough lurch, I lose last night's bluefish. What a start to the trip! Louis tells me that we're also having gear trouble; the automatic bilge pump is constantly running. I get into the cupboard under the sink where the pump sits, and manage to unblock it. It pumps for another minute and then stops, as it should when the automatic switch detects that there is no more bilge water. That's a great relief. It looks a wildly unsuitable set up for a bilge pump. A diaphragm pump with far too fine a strainer is calculated to block up and remain on automatic, pumping nothing.

The weather is uncomfortable but not life threatening. Twenty knots of wind would make a fine afternoon's sail, but the seas are steep because of the wind-against-current and getting any closer to beating would be very uncomfortable. The fog is a little thinner, but the cold is the main problem. I check the chart plotter and the chart. Still oceans of ocean in all directions. We're well past the meteorological buoy, and there's nowt else to hit save for any shipping. I decide that I'd better get some more rest while the other two are up. Breakfast has dropped off the agenda. I'm back asleep in minutes.

CHAPTER 25

Wet, wet, wet

19TH JUNE 2005

Scarlet is going like a bat out of hell. Having never sailed her in any kind of wind, we are impressed. The sea is heavy. We sail close-reached across a big swell but she just bounces along the black, confused sea. Let me at it, she seems to say.

The four-gallon, plastic water jars break loose again from where Louis has tied them and jog across the saloon. Two split open, adding streams of fresh water to the salty swirl. Louis dives under the dining table to tie the containers more securely and emerges with a face that is pale green. It is catching. When one person feels sick it infects everyone else. Or maybe the rolling sea and freezing fog are explanation enough. Or putting one's head under a table. Anyway – we are all feeing sick now.

Stef is the first to throw up. That's one fish supper over the railings. Scarlet races along at 10 knots straight into the wind, unconcerned that the entire crew is about to be very ill indeed.

The three of us sit in a row on deck in our foul weather gear, our mouths clamped shut. Stef and Louis have both given their fish suppers back to the fishes and I make the mistake of telling them that fishing is a very bad idea. Stupid to start an argument when you feel this horrible. We daren't open our mouths.

After a few hours I go below and cook plain pasta in chicken stock, the simplest thing I can think of for seasick, hungry, cold sailors. Only Stef swallows some. I can't manage even a spoonful but try a few blueberries, a spoonful of plain yoghurt and two dried apricots. Very soon, over the railings go: pasta in chicken stock, blueberries in yoghurt, two dried apricots.

Feeling this sick is all consuming.

Over the next three days and three nights we are able to eat nothing. I mean, nothing. We can barely manage to keep down a few sips of water. I have never felt this seasick in my life, and certainly not for days on end. I worry that we are all getting dehydrated; I know we have quickly become very weak. I have lost so much weight that my trousers won't stay up and I can see my ribs. God help Louis who was wafer thin before we set off.

Some time in the afternoon I surface. The wind and sea are both on the increase. The fog is thinner. Our course is even more south, no better than south east. The crew is even more wet. The bilge is full of water and soon the automatic bilge pump is back to its tricks. I try unblocking it but this time it's not having any. I search in vain for the switch to isolate it, but there doesn't appear to be one. Louis finds out how to disconnect it by pulling out a connector. I start manually pumping the bilge while trying to figure out where all this water is coming from. When the water level is down, I check the sea cocks.

Lynn announces that water has been trickling on to her berth in the fo'c'sle and that the underside of her mattress is soaking wet. It's a five inch thick mattress so it has taken a while for this to be evident. The first assumption is that water is still getting in through the dorades, so I check in the bedding cupboard, but there's no water in there now. Just wet sheets and towels. I can see the ventilator where the dorades enter and there's no water coming in there. Smothering by plastic bag is working. So where is it getting in? I must have pumped out at least thirty gallons.

Stef pumps out the bilge. Repeatedly. Each time he emerges from the bowels of the boat, he throws up – heavens know what because his stomach is achingly empty.

We are cold, wet, and sticky with salt. The bilge pump is broken. By beating into wind we encourage the leaks. We are down to one dry bunk between the three of us. The forward cabin is unusable, as is the big settee with the plinth in the middle. Bedding, pillows, duvets and clothes are all wet where water has poured into the lockers and cupboards. In the galley, even the cutlery and tea towels, kept in the top drawer, lie in inches of water. In the saloon, one window drips steadily down the food cupboard and onto the round settee. One cabin, two berths and our saloon are now no-go areas. We paddle around bare foot in the slopping water. From now on, we move in and out of the one dry berth like a game of musical chairs except there are no chairs and no music because we dare not waste the battery on the stereo. There is one dry pillow and one dirty, only slightly wet sheet.

We're going too fast. Lynn disengages the wind vane and heads us up nearer to wind while Louis and I put in another two reefs. That's us fully reefed now so the only option left is to lower the mainsail completely but it shouldn't come to that. The genoa is rolled down to a third. Scarlet wallows a fair bit when her bows are tucked into the sea but she seems comfortable enough, even if we're not. The cold and the wet are much more problematic than the state of the sea or the bilge pump. We're back to our reaching course now, as close to the wind as we can get without shipping too much over the bow, and doing a steady 8 knots, though steady is the last word I should use. The chart plotter says we're headed more or less straight at Bermuda which is not ideal. It is uncannily as if Scarlet heard that Bermuda was the original plan, and she is sticking to it. I tell her firmly that that was plan A and this is plan B, and we're supposed to be going straight across, not to Bermuda. We really don't want to be pushed too far south because what happens, as I read in *Ocean Passages*, is that the nor'easter then spits you out and dumps you in the calm of a Bermuda high.

CHAPTER 26

The Gulf Stream

21ST JUNE 2005

In this sorry state, sick, soaked and demoralised, we hit the Gulf Stream and the temperature suddenly rises. And rises. More water comes in. Louis and Stef are sharing the Captain's double bunk but I have decamped to the bench settee opposite the soaking wet one. The bench settee is OK on starboard tack because you are wedged up against the ceiling (for non-sailors that means the wall; don't ask me why), but on port tack I get thrown onto the floor.

The sea is like water in a washing machine because we have a NE wind and a very strong NE Gulf Stream current. Winds are named for where they come from. Currents from where they go to. Scarlet ploughs on, up to the top of a wave and scooshes down the undertow; up again, hover, crash; up, hover, crash.

Whereas a day ago I could not stop shivering, now it is so hot I am streaming sweat. Out on deck, Louis is wearing underpants and an anorak. I try to cook but am thrown straight across the cabin to land whack against the opposite wall. I can wedge my back against the engine cupboard when I am right in front of the cooker, but when I move an inch or two sideways away from this snug backrest, to the sink or to the work surface, there is nothing to hold me so I am jettisoned across the cabin and dumped on the floor on the other side. I feel so damn sick and now I am covered in bruises. My arms are taking the brunt of this fairground ride because instinctively I hold them out to break the crash into the next hard object.

We move through huge seas and stir-crazy waves. Stef and I eat the odd morsel and promptly throw up. Louis just doesn't eat. The watch system falls apart. Whoever feels least bad at any time is on duty. The other two try to sleep, usually wedged together in the same bunk.

My memory all goes a bit mushy here. The on and off of watches crosscuts the day and night – light and dark. I clearly remember waking in my bunk when Louis is on watch and feeling that the boat's motion has changed, and feeling warmer as we suddenly enter the Gulf Stream and begin to bounce across the steeper waves. Like everything else, Scarlet is taking it in her stride so I go back to sleep. When I next wake and talk to Louis, he tells me how definite the transition was, the water changing colour as we hit warmth. I didn't see it but I didn't miss it either because the change in the motion was just as definite when I was half asleep in my bunk. Some monitoring bit of my mind knew the place we had sailed into because I dreamt vivid colours of pale green and purple.

The mind works differently out on the deep sea where not just memory plays tricks but also the imaginary geography. However homogeneous the sea is, my mind develops its own geography which is always out of sight, but carves our course for us. Arriving at the Gulf Stream is as definite an event as arriving at a cross roads. When we eventually get into the steady westerlies across the 40th parallel, it feels as if we're sailing beside a highway that is just over the horizon. When the wind shifts our course even a few degrees I sense that we're straying off a path that is as tangible as a path in the forest, all felt through the change in the angle of boat to wave.

What I don't remember at all is eating. Drinking is mandated by considered knowledge that dehydration kills but I don't remember eating more than half a cereal bar for a couple of days in this first half-gale, and here the memory is right I suspect.

The day after the night when we crossed into the Gulf Stream, things quieten down. The wind is down to perhaps 17 knots, and it's even relented a shade north allowing us to make a bit better than south east. The sea is down a little, though still strong enough to stop any consideration of hardening up to further improve our course, at least while we are taking on water. The genoa is out to two-thirds, we have shaken a couple of reefs out of the main, and it's blessedly warm. Oh what a relief to get out of the fog and the cold. Remind me not to go high latitude sailing! I have to pump the bilge by hand again, emptying another thirty gallons, but now we can take stock.

The weather has been kind to a captain and crew who mistimed their exit. The effect of the wind blowing against the Gulf Stream could have been very much worse. It blew no more than gusts of 30 knots, and mostly 20–25 which would have been ideal for an afternoon sail when sea-legs had been found, leaks eliminated, and the boat had become familiar. We are sorely missing our two week shakedown cruise, and I take my hat off to delivery skippers who pick up unknown boats and set off into the blue. Some fog was to be expected, though I underestimated how cold it would be. I also underestimated how much trouble we would have close reaching into a 15–20 knot north-easter which was pushing us south. We were promised N backing NW, but given N veering NE.

But the real problem is the leaking. I have made several bad mistakes. I should have gone to much greater lengths to plug the hawse pipe before we set off, but had not wanted to pull Louis away from enjoying the departure. Then I should have spent more effort getting to grips with the problem when we did start taking on water. Feeling cold is much exacerbated by being wet. My brain doesn't work well when cold and wet and anxious about essentials like the bilge pump. Louis had a look in the anchor locker in the forepeak to see if the water was getting in through the hawse pipe because that was obviously hypothesis number one. There was water coming in but hardly enough to account for the inflow. All our previous boats, and every other one I had heard of, have anchor lockers that drain out straight into the sea. Even though this boat is much larger, its anchor locker drain seems to go into the bilge. Perhaps a one inch drain hole in the bow offended someone's sensibilities? Accurate diagnosis is tricky at present with the bow burying itself every twenty seconds or so.

I pull up the wet fo'c'sle mattresses and lift the lids to the stowage space beneath. It's very hard to trace what happens at the bottom of the space beneath the anchor locker but there appears to be a pipe which is probably intended to take the water draining back to the bilge. This pipe is inaccessible for most of its length but appears to be blocked and the water is seeping back under the floor and sternward into the bilge. I can't think where else the water can be coming in. Louis valiantly does another wet cold stint on the foredeck with some plastic sheet and cable ties, and manages to throttle the hawse pipe. It's designed in such a way that it's very hard to plug up. This seems to have the desired effect down below. A few drips are getting in but these are tolerable.

That night on my watch I see the first shipping since we set out. A couple of big container ships, perhaps an hour apart, on the same heading, in the sea lane into New York. They're far enough away that they never look like bothering us. I feel they are company but at the same time a warning that we're not away from human hazards yet.

CHAPTER 27

Alternative alternators

We have been charging the batteries by running the engine for an hour a day. Some alternative source of electricity is high on our list of desirables, but that's for later. The battery monitor system, which I'm just beginning to understand, shows that the batteries are low, lower than they should be. All we're using is navigation lights and periodical electronics and cabin lights.

After breakfast – yes eating has resumed – I start the engine to find there is no current going into the batteries. I hinge the forward companionway steps up, take the front box off the engine, and straightaway can see why. There are bits of belt and black rubber powder all over. The alternator belt is shredded as well as one of the doubled-up fridge compressor belts. I brought three spare alternator belts, so this in itself is not serious, but there is the question: Why? It could be that the alternator belt just broke and took the much heavier compressor belt with it, or vice versa. We don't have a spare compressor belt because it is a nonstandard belt which I couldn't buy off the shelf in Newport. The double is still there, but if it breaks under the extra load and takes another alternator belt, that would not be good.

Louis and I dig out the tool box and a spare alternator belt. Changing a car alternator belt can be fairly straightforward but here there is a mass of stuff on the front of the engine that has to come off: the cooling water pump and hoses, the fridge compressor, and so on. Louis and I each work out a sequence of disassembly and compare notes. Our plans agree, as they usually do on these occasions. One tricksy part is that the cooling water hose is below sea level and so will start letting in ocean when we have disconnected it. We dig out a plug. We're about to find out the state of corrosion of all the screws, clips, nuts and bolts. Some further digging reveals that the reason the belt broke is that the bracket that holds it out from the engine, and so holds the belt tight, has broken right off the engine block. The weld has cracked and there's no prospect of welding it back while at sea. This is a bit disconcerting. No alternator, no electricity. The most serious loss will be the navigation lights. It looks as if it should be possible to jury rig an arrangement whereby the body of the alternator is pulled out away from the block with some cord passed around a strong point on the engine frame. This should be OK because the frame is integral with the engine and should vibrate in synch with it, rather than tearing itself to pieces when the engine vibrates relative to the boat. Louis finds some good strong nylon cord and a carabiner which will provide a chafe free attachment point.

We set to work disassembling, and an hour later we have the new belt on and jury rigged. There will be a lot of force on the belt because the batteries are down and the alternator is a heavy-duty marine one producing the best part of 100 amps. Cross fingers and fire her up. I go on deck to flick the switch. Louis shouts up that it looks good. I duck into the rear cabin and see the red LEDs on the battery monitor are lit. There's 80 amps going into the battery. This is heart warming in the extreme. I confess to a certain obsessiveness about the care and feeding of batteries and their sources of juice, nurtured by a long career of old cars and boats with rickety electricity supplies. A full battery, or even a positive reading on an ammeter, makes the heart glow. Back down at the engine, Louis pronounces it good. There's not too much vibration, so the string seems to be doing its stuff. Not the most reassuring set up in the early part of a transatlantic crossing, but we're not going to abandon ship just yet.

Stef makes it all sound so matter-of-fact. When the engine breaks its fan belt, my husband and son spend half a day sliding around on their bums, naked except for knickers, painting the cabin sole with black greasy hand and foot prints. If they can't mend the fan belt (or whatever) we will have no lights, including no navigation lights. After four hours they get it going again with a piece of string. They inform me the string could snap in ten minutes or in an hour or next week.

Keeping one's cool! The next decision is the fridge/freezer. The system can run off the mains in dock, or off the compressor on the engine at sea, but it doesn't run off the 12v battery supply. There's no dock in sight. We could risk running it off the engine on a single belt, but if the belt breaks, it'll probably take the alternator belt with it and may do damage to our other rather delicate lashings. We have two more spare alternator belts, and I even bought a spare alternator. Being without electricity altogether would not be funny. We have enough dry cell batteries to run Gecko – the backup GPS – for about three months, but we'd have no navigation lights. The world band radio will work on dry cell batteries but the weather fax needs the laptop, and the laptop needs the ship's batteries. If we used nothing else, the laptop would run for quite a while on the 400 ampere hours of a full set of ship's batteries. But they are not really full.

It looks like no fridge and no freezer. Lynn will not be happy. They're reasonably well insulated, but there's a lot of cold stuff in there which won't stay cold for more than a couple of days. An awful lot of food must either be eaten, or fed to the fishes. Good job we are over the sea sickness. We start on *la grand bouffe*. All the goodies and perishables first. We won't get scurvy for a few days.

The wind is dropping. By a nice irony, the genoa furling line frays through. The past few days of blow, with it partly furled, have been too much for it. Of course, it frays at the roller so that neither half of the line is long enough to function, and it's not possible to join it any way that will go through all the fairleads. It looks as if the angle of entry of the line onto the furling drum is not adjusted quite right, and the result is chafe. For now, it's foredeck work to adjust the genoa using half a broom handle as a makeshift winch.

Louis keeps announcing flying fish. They shoot out of the sides of waves and skitter thirty yards across the surface before plunging in again, hoping that the beast that hunts beneath has been thrown off their trail. Most of them are so fast that you only see them out of the corner of your eye. Announcements are, by their nature, of flying fish past and buried. Lynn is tormented by her failure to see them and suspects her son is winding her up. I catch enough out of the corner of my eye to assure her he is not.

CHAPTER 28

⚓

Becalmed

We are wallowing about. We are becalmed with the sun on full beam. We've predictably been spat out the north-easter into the Bermuda high. We celebrate the end of the blow by hanging everything wet over the rails until we look like a gypsy encampment. Even the fo'c'sle mattresses are out on deck. The crew is also laid out to dry.

Since we're right down to half a knot, we decide on a swim, first trailing a line over the bow, the full length of the boat and out astern. A fender tied horizontally beneath the gate through the rails on the quarter serves as a boarding ladder. Louis jumps in from the pulpit with a scream and an earsplitting grin. The captain has some of a sailor's reticence about swimming, but even he takes a dip. Lynn is slightly more conservative and instead of her usual immediate dash for the horizon, she seems fond of the rope, and not fond of the news, which, after consulting the chart, is that the water is about four miles deep. The water is curiously clear and blue, almost sterile. There are odd bits of weed, the yellow side of seaweed green, which we dub Neptune's Bath Sponge. We've already spotted Portuguese men of war floating past, so a strict jellyfish watch is kept by those on deck when anyone is in the water. The first mate is a bit paranoid about them. I wonder to myself what the Portuguese call them; Jellypesce Ingles?

Louis announces that he is going swimming. The Atlantic, Stef tells us, is four miles deep, and we are a thousand miles from land with only the horizon for company. I consider this information for a while but decide to pretend it's just another swim off the boat somewhere near land. I want a swim but I don't want to freak out; self-deception is therefore the solution. Louis walks up to the prow and jumps in, a grin on his face. I have the camera in my hand so the moment with him in midair is captured forever. While he swims, I stand guard for Portuguese Man o' War which have been drifting past our boat in a steady procession. They look like shimmering poly bags with nasty little sails above the water which point this way and that in the wind, their poisonous tentacles hanging treacherously below the surface.

'It's the clearest, warmest water I have ever swum in,' yells a spluttery voice from the ocean.

We rig up a rope so that those of us who are sensible (me) can swim with it looped around an ankle. Others can risk getting separated from the boat and floating away towards the horizon if they wish but since we have no engine, separation seems like a bad idea. The surprise is the temperature of the water. You would expect a four-mile deep ocean to be icy cold, but it is warm. Gentle and warm. I swim round and round the boat while Stef takes up jellyfish watch. Getting out is more difficult than getting in but with a fender hung longways over the side, I can just about haul myself up having got one foot on the rubber step. While Louis and I sun ourselves, Stef swims. He is less traumatised by jellyfish than we are.

Later, while I am asleep, and Louis is alone on watch, he sees a fair sized turtle swimming close to the boat.

I have really enjoyed today. And saying this I can admit that I have not enjoyed many of the other days. Or hours. The boat is drying out, something I would not have thought possible. Louis has been able to move back into his forward cabin, still a bit damp, but usable, and that satisfies my maternal need for him to be comfortable and to have some degree of privacy. In the evening we sit on deck to watch the sunset and wolf down pasta with smoked sausage and Swiss cheese. Things taste wonderful when you are at sea and hungry.

After the dip, I decide it would be useful to have some weather information. Louis has been making periodic attempts at getting the Sony world band to pick up one or other of the forecasts listed in Reed's Almanac but without any audible luck. We decide on a concerted go at the weather fax, fetching the radio and the laptop out on deck, along with the list of station wavelengths. We can pick up the fax signals where they are predicted by the wavelengths, and the dongle seems to be decoding them into something that the software vaguely recognises. This looks promising. We get something that is speckled with noise but has isobars on it, and what looks like the Chesapeake is just about interpretable. Extending the wire aerial doesn't help as much as I'd hoped. We try hoisting the wire up the flag halyard so that it's vertical. No better. A crocodile clip connection on the backstay improves the signal noticeably. We get something that looks like the iceberg forecast, but without icebergs. But then there shouldn't be any icebergs.

It's puzzling that the reception isn't better. This is a powerful government station transmitting from somewhere near Boston and I would expect it to produce a close to optimal signal. After huge amounts of permuting of arrangements, we finally get something that is a legible fax, with just one peculiarity; it is split down the middle with the left half on the right, and the right on the left. We read the manual several times for ways of correcting this. It has corrections for a number of derangements but not this one. This turns out to be the best fax we manage for the entire trip. Probably the aerial is at fault so later we will have to look into different aerial systems, but for this trip we're down to VHF pleadings to passing ships as far as weather information is concerned.

I was foolish to rely on the broker's statements that we had an SSB and the salesman's statement that we would get a satellite connection, but even more foolish not to take the time to test out the weather fax system before leaving.

Despite the warmth of the sun and the luxurious swim, the crew is still demoralised. Lynn particularly is understandably unhappy about the boat being so wet. Louis thinks the communication arrangements are RUBBISH. He's right of course.

Chapter 29

Father and son

Stef and Louis spend the whole day mending broken bits of equipment, patching sails, securing things with ropes, pushing more polythene bags into the places which leak. They are both exhausted. They work slowly and only because they have to. There is no joy in the completion of tasks and their usual silent or jokey companionship is taut and strained.

I worry continuously because my son is ill now and struggling, yet he continues to do heroic stuff to help his father and to pull his weight – of which there is not much left. I can see his ribs and shoulder blades sharp and spare and his trousers fall down from a waist most women would die for. I don't want my son to die from a twenty inch waist. I write with black humour, but what I feel is deep maternal guilt and tearful despair. When you have ME, you have to preserve your energy, not throw yourself into a vortex that sucks the living daylights out of you. I fear for my son. Stef and I wanted to do this. If we suffer, so be it. But we pressured Louis to come with us and he does not deserve, nor can he cope, with much more.

This evening Louis and I go into a worried, mutinous huddle. One quick exchanged look and we know that it is crunch time. We are too weak to coil a rope and we move about the boat in slow motion. To continue with a crew this unwell would be dangerous and foolhardy. What is more, we are both aware that our skipper has started to behave oddly. He seems to have drifted away from us and detached himself into his own world. He has gone silent, something he does only when pushed to his limits. Much of the time he appears catatonic, passing hours sitting on deck staring at the sea. I have seen him behave like this for short periods, after some crisis, but never for a whole day.

'He's gaga,' Louis says. 'He doesn't know what he's doing.'

'He goes silent when he's really worried, and exhausted.

'He's not doing anything. Just staring into space. I'm making the decisions, not him.'

'I know. Thank heavens you are here.'

It's true. Stef looks utterly spaced out. So it falls to Louis to monitor the situation and to somehow keep a clear head. There is far too much pressure on my son; far too much for his young shoulders to carry.

We confront Stef together. We tell him, if conditions are no better in the morning, we have to head for Bermuda. Of course he opposes the idea and, in his present bizarre mental state which seems not to admit reality or reason, he can only see plan A. We are going to the Canaries.

'It's too late to change course,' he argues. 'Hurricane season.'

'The boat us heading for Bermuda,' Louis insists. 'We should stay on this course.'

'It's land. We can reach it before we all collapse,' I add. 'Apart from Bermuda there is nothing. We are not well enough to continue to the Canaries. Please listen.'

They stage a mutiny. We want to go to Bermuda, they chorus. I point out that whereas Bermuda was a sensible plan when we had two weeks more than we now have. It is late in the season and it is not clear how helpful it would be. We would then face the problem of getting back to the east coast. Leaving the boat in Bermuda is not an option because of the VAT which we would have to pay there. It would ruin us.

However, they aren't budging so the captain decides to capitulate rather than casting himself off in the dinghy.

Stef is appalled, crestfallen, shocked but we tell him 'crew before course' to which there is no reply. But I know he is not really listening, certainly not agreeing, and he will do anything to wriggle out of this change of plan. My husband is stubborn. Right now, he is half crazy with the conditions we have been through – and stubborn. He will not admit defeat.

We change course southward although at our snail's pace this is more of an intention than an achievement of a change of position. Although nothing but the compass needle in the binnacle and the heading read-out on the chart-plotter change, it feels completely different pointing this way, and I don't like it.

We try a series of exhausting tacks. We can't get east. Can't get south east. We try tacking the other way. No better.

Again Louis and I approach our tightlipped, blank-faced skipper to tell him that our decision of the previous night remains unchanged.

'Look, we are both exhausted,' I say, when I can get his attention. 'We have no stamina and no strength left. It is dangerous to continue with a crew in this state.'

Still he refuses to admit the severity of the situation, and for a few minutes argues every which way about imminent hurricanes, the fact that Bermuda is a 'dead-end' and the fact that we have not paid VAT on the boat.

'Well, if you want to give up, we might as well turn back to the east coast, right?' Stef says.

'It's not a question of giving up, it's a question of survival,' I counter. 'From here, the obvious course is to head for Bermuda. There is no point in turning around and heading back.'

We continue to argue about the merits of Bermuda versus turning back through the seas that have nearly finished us off when Louis loses his rag.

'I'm fucking exhausted. OK?' He shouts.

It doesn't come plainer than that.

My husband is clever at bending reality to fit what he wants to believe, but he cannot deny the difficulties of the past three days, nor can he fail to see that his crew are in bad shape. Finally, and with very bad grace, he concedes defeat because it involves taking no action and perhaps that is the only reason he agrees. We continue on the same course because it happens to be right course for Bermuda.

We travel to Bermuda for exactly three hours. At least in my head I believe that we are travelling to Bermuda even if we are sailing the very same track as before. But Stef continues to worry out loud about the hurricane season and the fact that we have no insurance cover for Bermuda. He is sitting on deck with his mouth all grim and his head furrowed. He isn't speaking to us except to say that even if we get there safely, which in his opinion is unlikely, we will have to move on again almost straightaway. We say we don't care. We are going to Bermuda. He is not happy. I am happy because I am soon going to get off this soaking wet bloody boat and my son will get a rest. Louis and I go below to get away from the angry skipper and to find Bermuda on the chart plotter and point the little virtual orange boat in that direction. I manage to eat half a biscuit.

The skipper remains in a black, bleak mood. After a couple more hours of sulking and grim silence in the cockpit, he says – like this is news – 'Trying to get to Bermuda is fucking dangerous, right! We can't rule out sailing straight into a hurricane.'

Here we go again. We've been round this garden path at least ten times.

'It would help if we had some means of getting some weather information,' Louis points out dryly.

'And how would that help?'

'We can sail the other way if we know a hurricane is coming.'

Stupid! I add under my breath.

'You think that will save you!'

'It might have been sensible to make sure we had weather information before setting off,' Louis says, not for the first or last time.

This little conversation is a leitmotif which will drift on throughout our trip. Fortunately the technology side of things was, with their complete agreement, their department, so it's not my fault!

At about 2 p.m., Stef takes a decision which amazes me.

'We're going to head back to the east coast,' he announces. 'It's madness going to Bermuda.'

My daring, unflappable husband is giving in. Never in all my years of sailing with him have I heard him admit defeat. Always it has been:

We should just about make it.

We'll just inch over the sandbar.

Take the sails down; we'll ride it out.

Let's keep going. We should get there by nightfall.
In shocked silence, we change course for the Chesapeake.

By evening we're not much nearer Bermuda, if at all. We can't keep tacking all the way to Bermuda. We're making no headway. I decide that the only option is to turn back to the Chesapeake. One week into our crossing and we are only three hundred miles from our starting point and the crew is defeated.

LOUIS

I don't remember anything like this much discussion. Dad was definitely
out of it. Mum and I were very ill. But Mum's account is how I remember
it.

CHAPTER 30

⚓

Back to the Chesapeake

23RD JUNE 2005

I'm slightly happier with this full Uey, but only slightly. One of our earlier plans had been to leave the boat over there, or perhaps even a bit further south where the winters are milder and the need to be in a shed less compelling. On the other hand I still don't like it. I can see the argument that at our present speed it will take two months to get to the Azores, but we aren't going to stay at this speed. Lynn and Louis have been very stoic to get this far without caving in.

We turn round and spend the night sailing back towards the Chesapeake. The wind picks up and the ceiling comes down, and we're broad reaching at a good clip, around 5 to 6 knots. I do a long watch knowing that the other two are done in. The temperature is perfect although the lowering cloud and the shift of course brings on a slight feeling of foreboding. I doze on and off and spend the night stretched out across the seat behind the helm which is inch perfect for me.

In my mental maritime geography I am sailing to Texas. Don't ask me why Texas, or even how I know that it's Texas, but it's a vivid sensation. Perhaps the wind vane has decided to go home? Perhaps it's because I once drove across Oklahoma all night to the Texas panhandle, and it wasn't a lot more featureful than this bit of ocean. Anyway, it is Texas we are heading for, a good deal south of the Chesapeake, but I suppose the bearing wouldn't be all that different at this distance. I should look on the chart and work it out. I suspect this state of mind is sparked by the involuntary change of course rumbling around my psyche.

The wind is on the nose as we try to cross the confused currents of the Gulf Stream. In twenty-four hours we travel twelve nautical miles towards the States. The current pulls one way; Scarlet tries to push the other. We try motoring but after four hours we have traveled a mile. In a state of self-deception, I feel more settled and secure in the knowledge that we are, in theory, heading for dry land, albeit the land we set out from a week ago. Two more days of this, I keep telling myself, counting the hours and mentally crossing them off, then a marina. A shower. Dry clothes. No rocking motion.

At 8 a m, Lynn wakes me up and chides me gently for my substandard watch keeping. At noon the chart-plotter indicates that since we changed course we have made about 15 miles in 12 hours while moving at an average of 5 knots through the water. When I agreed to go along with the mutiny, I did believe that the new course was a possible option but now we must be back in a Gulf Stream running at around 3.5 knots. We spend the rest of the day setting various courses across the stream while trying to get log and chart-plotter to agree on the direction and speed of the current. The data is all over the place. Our best course seems to be a little north of direct. Later, when we are closer to the coast, we can, of course, get back down on the back eddy which runs down the coast. Of course we can. Or am I trying to reassure myself?

Unable to find a good course in all these eddies, Louis and I start a more minute inspection of the June planning chart which shows the wind direction and statistics, and the direction and speed of the current for the north Atlantic. On the laptop we can blow up the relevant section between Bermuda and the coast. It looks more diffuse than it does on the Admiralty chart, and my memory of the planning chart has the Gulf Stream current continuing north east much further into the coast. The currents are less intense than the Gulf Stream proper, but quite enough to be troublesome – 3 knots in places. Louis and I begin to be concerned that we could be going up the down escalator, and we could remain on the down escalator fighting the Gulf Stream and its offshoots and eddies all the way back to the Chesapeake.

⚓

CHAPTER 31

If only Captain Bligh had been the patient type

25TH JUNE 2005

It's three days since we made the decision to give up on the crossing and sail back to the Chesapeake but we have been blown further and further south and are now well below Newport where we began. The accepted way to cross the Atlantic is to head for the Forties, pick up the prevailing wind, and blow across in an elegant arc. What we have done is to sail round in one huge half circle ending up three hundred miles further south than we should be, as helpless as a paper boat in a vortex, the Gulf Stream clinging on to us while Scarlet is blown further and further south.

4 p.m.

Stef and Louis are having an earnest discussion on deck. I know what this is about, and I don't want to hear it. Finally they call me up and confront me.

'We have an impossible decision to make,' Louis says. 'Either we continue like this, perhaps for another week, trying to get across the Gulf Stream, or we turn around again and head for the Azores.'

That's what I thought they were talking about.

'How far to the Azores?' I ask.

'Two thousand miles.'

We discuss the three options:

1. We continue on the present course towards the Chesapeake with unfavourable northerly winds and the current against us.
2. We sail further north, back to Long Island.
3. We turn around (again) and head for Europe.

We debate the first two options with me silently praying for the resolution I favour. However, the charts reveal that the westerly current of the Gulf Stream fans out further north than we originally thought with only a narrow strip of counter current along the coast. We would have the same kind of trouble heading north as trying to head west. The patterns and flows of the current suggest that it could take another week to claw our way north only to be spat out – in Ferry Cove Boatworks!

The crew is beat. I want to get back to land.

The Skipper says, 'Even if we make landfall eventually, how will we feel catching a plane home after a completely abortive trip? What will this do for our morale, our feelings about the boat, our future sailing plans?'

I know that Stef and Louis have already decided. They are just waiting for my agreement and, looking at their sober faces, I understand that I have no choice but to trust their judgment.

'OK,' I say.

They look relieved. Louis gives me a wet hug.

'That's brave,' he says.

Later Louis comes and sits beside me below deck.

'Do we have enough food?' he asks.

My poor son, ill with ME, is always ravenous, always suffering stomach pains. He seems unable to take nutrition from what he eats and so is constantly anxious about low blood sugar and its horrible consequences. Food supplies have concerned him, I suspect, more than storms and hurricanes. We have used up a week's supplies and are still in Square One on the ocean game board. No, it's worse than that – we have not even reached Square One. I sit down with my notepad. I make an inventory of all the food we have left and make a list of meals, catering for the worst case scenario of a trip of three more weeks to reach the Azores.

'We can do it,' I tell him, 'if you don't mind lots of rice and pasta.'

'I need protein,' he tells me. 'One-third of a tin of tuna is not enough for me.'

'You can have my third.'

'Still not enough. I need two tins.'

I know. Protein is what his body needs to work at all. To be honest, we do not have much protein as in fresh steak and lamb stew and chickens roasting on a spit but we do have cheese and beef jerky, and I suppose he might catch another fish.

'I think we'll manage,' I tell him.

He looks very doubtful. I feel very doubtful.

It's late afternoon, and we're going nowhere. We are lined up three in a row on the windward cockpit seat. At 36 degrees 45' north, 69 degrees 54' west, at 17.15, we turn for the Azores.

We celebrate the decision by executing a perfect gybe – our first in Scarlet – and head north to get back into the westerlies. *Ocean Passages* assures us that these westerlies start at 40 degrees north, and that coming from Bermuda it is worth the detour to get up north to 40 degrees, rather than trying to cut the corner north east across the Bermuda High. After gybing, we immediately feel better. We're back trying to do what we set out to do. The boat feels happier and picks up a brisk 6 knots.

What day is it? We think the 25th but we're not sure.

CHAPTER 32

First Time Spinnaker

Of course the wind doesn't last.

The next day it fades so much that we decide to get the spinnaker out. The extent of our spinnaker experience is not great and we haven't even looked inside the bag at the one on this boat. We had one on the boat before last, but it didn't get much use because the crew wasn't yet beefy enough. We time ourselves at one hour, ten minutes, twenty-two seconds to get it up. The twelve meter crew back in Newport would be unhappy at twenty-two seconds but they have done it before and there are twelve of them.

We are pleased with ourselves and the big sail pulls nicely. Lynn even approves of the powder blue and white against our dark blue hull. A colour clash could have been serious. The spinnaker gives us a couple of extra knots from our two knot baseline. We have had to jury rig a down-haul having not quite sussed out where all the bits and pieces go. Later, this down-haul proves difficult to untie, so we are left with a line clove-hitched around the spinnaker pole for a while until I soak it off a few days later. The joys of an unfamiliar boat!

Another morning, and it is a broiler with not a whisper of wind. Undeterred, the Skipper Who Never Admits To No Wind tells us to raise the spinnaker. I've not even seen it yet, but now, aided by the keen pair on deck, here it comes spilling out of its bag, a slippery, chiffony mass of tissue paper fabric with blue and white stripes. When it is up and filled with wind it looks like a squashed rugby ball, but I am getting way ahead of myself. It comes encased in a snuffer – a huge condom which is pulled up to release the sail, and quickly (in theory) dropped down again to extinguish it when you realise a gale is about to strike. When the spinnaker is out – and a spectacular sight it is – the snuffer sits on top like Wee Willie Winkie's hat. I had forgotten the palaver of raising a spinnaker. First the massive spinnaker pole has to be taken off the mast where it is stored in an upright position and dragged (with much cursing and huffing and puffing from the skipper who always accompanies physical effort with sympathetic verbal accompaniment) until it lies horizontal on deck with its tip sticking out over the prow. Then you burrow into the balloon of fabric to find and identify the three corners to be attached to the pole and the correct ropes. It is very easy to get it all screwed up with the left rope on the right side, and so on, which of course Stef and Louis do several times. Sailors, please forgive this long description, but I want others to know what is involved in raising and dousing a football pitch-sized sail.

It takes them nearly one and a half hours to raise the spinnaker for the first time. Stef says the crew of a racing twelve meter can do it in thirty-five seconds so they have a way to go.

We spinnaker across the wide flat blue sea for the rest of the day

10 p.m.
Louis has worked like a dog today so Stef and I offer to split his night shift between us, but after an hour or so the spinnaker is tying itself in knots around its pole and we have to summon him from his bed. Because I took no part in putting up the spinnaker, I am of no assistance dousing it.

The two men go up on deck. Without a moon it is pitch black with the boat set against complete darkness. I can see them in silhouette moving around in the white beam from the torch and the red glow from Louis's little miner's head lamp. It is like modern dance; two men in bright blue harnesses and the enormous blue-striped spinnaker against a black stage set. If it weren't for the fear of one or both of them falling overboard as they grapple with the tissue fabric, I could just sit here all night and watch the surreal performance. For a second, one face is lit. Then a torso. The red light beams upwards and down again. Louis is lean and brown and naked under his cobalt harness. It is eerily beautiful, this slow ballet that is danced in red and white ribbons of light. If I were a choreographer, I would set it to Philip Glass.

At last the spinnaker is snuffed and bagged and they hoist the mainsail. 'Very slick,' says Stef when they finish. 'Text book stuff.'

'I wouldn't like to do it in any wind,' Louis says, and goes back to bed.

11 p.m.

An almighty clanging reaches into my dreams and jolts me awake. Why are we rolling as if in a giant swell? The clanging comes from the mast which is very close to my ear. Clang, bang, clang. I shout, 'Bloody hell!' because I do so want to sleep, and my long-suffering son emerges from his cabin for the second time tonight. Clang. Bang. Pause of exactly three seconds. Clang. Bang. The three of us are on deck now, rubbing sleepy eyes. We agree that there is not a whisper of wind, but cannot find the source of the clanging so we agree to lower the mainsail and let Scarlet drift for the night.

Midnight.

Louis returns to bed for the third time. My nerves are so frayed from the clanging noise that my legs are jerking and twitching, and my heart has gone into overdrive – bangabangabang.

A wallowy night follows. There are urgent and pitiful pleadings from below that I do something to stop the rolling. Like put my leg out and extend it the full three miles down.

CHAPTER 33

Up the mast

Another day, another lull. But remember that my husband is one of those sailors who swears that there is no such thing as no wind.

But back to the end of last night's watch. The sails begin blowing about in an irritating way, hanging loose, then twitching from one side to the other. After fiddling with the wind vane, pulling first its left string, then its right, I decide that either the wind is blowing in circles or it is dying. I have finally worked out a mnemonic for the wind vane which I repeat like a mantra before I adjust it: pull right string to go left; pull left string to go right. I don't know how the wonderful contraption works but this seems fairly foolproof. Stef says he pretends he is driving a bus backwards – which is really helpful! Anyway, no matter what I do to the strings, the sails flap. I can't see the instrument dials without a torch and I can't find the torch. Appalling seamanship! It is obvious that no-one has lived on this boat before; she needs pockets out on deck for torches and spectacles and mugs.

On cue, Stef pokes his head out. 'Wind gone?'

Even asleep or half-asleep, he never turns off his weather antennae and can detect a change in the wind of more than 10 degrees and/or a knot. Together we mess about with the wind vane and the sails for another hour until I pronounce the situation temporarily hopeless and go to bed. For the rest of the night Louis and I are shaken and tossed to the accompaniment of the clang of the boom bashing from side to side, the slapping of sails against the mast, the racket of the rigging.

Why doesn't he bloody give up and tie everything down and let us sleep!

Next morning we find out what all the banging was about. In the process of adjusting the mainsail I find that it's jammed at the head. A great deal of fiddling it up and down fails to free it. It looks like a trip up the mast is the only solution and Louis bravely volunteers. Perhaps he rates his chances at the top better than the chance of being landed on by his father accelerating sixty feet downward. He digs out the climbing harness bought especially for this contingency, clips on two halyards, puts one on the most powerful mast winch, and gives Lynn the other one to hold as a backup. Louis collects some tools and up he goes, me winching, he climbing, and Lynn taking up the slack on the safety.

First spreader, unlatch safety, re-latch safety.

Second spreader, same again.

He finds a raised screw head in the track right up near the top, catching the sail slide. Lynn ties off the safety line and becomes the camera crew. We have pictures of a very small fellah at the top of the mast, but they don't convey the true height or the rolling motion. Louis gets the screw bedded back down, and by the time he's finished seems to be quite enjoying himself up there.

Can't say I fancy it myself.

CHAPTER 34

⚓

Blue eggs

When I poke my head out at 7.30 a.m., jaded and ready to give my husband an earful for the sleepless night of boom noises, I see that the sky is a brilliant blue. The sea is flat-calm. There is absolutely no wind. I shut my mouth because suddenly life is worth living again.

Bleary and rheumy-eyed, I climb the steps of the companionway to see an ocean like an ironed blue sheet. Louis is swimming near the boat and Stef's naked body drips salt water into the cockpit. With a Mogadon hangover, I dare not jump in case I sink.

Louis shouts, 'Can't touch the bottom, even with my big toe!'

Caffeine is required, and toast, a breakfast more suited to a cold English city morning than this scorching seascape but that is all we have. It is already 100 degrees

I go back to bed and sleep heavily for three hours. When I wake again, Louis says he is hungry and Stef says Louis is hungry. I suggest omelettes (protein!) but the first two eggs out of the box are blue. We have our familiar family argument in which Stef asserts that anything not crawling is edible, and I say that salmonella on a boat is not a good idea. Blue eggs are not a good idea. Louis agrees with me. We break open more eggs. Another blue one. Then five yellow ones. Stef works out the statistics on three blue eggs followed by five yellow ones while I cook omelettes.

Lunch over, the men go back to their deck work while the boat is, for once, not a fairground ride. I pick up all the soaked clothes and bedding, wring them, and hang them over the rails. Dry salty clothes are better than wet salty clothes. I drag the foam mattresses through the hatches and prop them up to dry. I hang the duvets and duvet covers over the boom since it is out of commission. I clean out the forward head and bag up all the wet toilet rolls. We are a travelling launderette, steaming in the sun, and I am its satisfied manager, content that I can salvage something to wear and something to sleep on in the aftermath of living inside a washing machine for a week. My men folk continue to take off shackles, untangle sheets (the other sort), solve the jams and conundrums. We have reverted to stereotypical gender roles, them above deck doing 'men's work', me below picking up and cleaning, sorting and stowing, tidying and folding, wiping and drying.

Now that we are becalmed again, Louis worries that the food is going to run out while I worry for Louis that the food will run out. When I look inside the fridge and freezer to do a bit of stocktaking, what I see makes my heart sink for my poor hungry son. Our cold supplies swim in several inches of stinking water.

I chuck overboard:

Loads of uncooked croissants which have swelled and puffed out of their tins. They float in water like grotesque wet balloons.

Four packets of juice

Four large tubs of yoghurt

Four packets of cream

Blueberries

Chocolate, all pale with sea-water

Six packets of tortillas which have turned mottled blue.

I skim the tortillas over the water like flat stones.

I salvage: A few packets of Swiss cheese still sealed. Sealed smoked sausages.

I devise the following survival diet:

Don't eat the contents of the tins yet.

Eat the sausage and cheese until they grow mould – with pasta, with rice, with anything.

Louis is very worried. I think and plan and dream food from this day on.

The fridge contents are getting more dubious by the hour. Necessity invented mothers and so Lynn reinvents flapjack, or rather a cross between flapjack, muesli and granola. Vast quantities of almost rancid, past-sell-by-date butter are poured on to piles of porridge oats, flavoured with maple syrup, and stirred and stirred until the whole boat smells divine. We eat it with spoons out of bowls. This proves our staple magic dust for the rest of the trip, getting us out of all sorts of desponds.

After his dip, Louis has the energy to worry about food and survival and scurvy again – this is becoming his refrain and each new chorus produces maternal shame and guilt that my poor provisioning is a constant, nagging source of anxiety for him. He calculates that at a conservative average of 5 knots a day, it will take us another twenty-one days to reach the Azores.

Back I go to do another stocktaking and present them with a somewhat disheartening summary of our calorific situation:

Six two-gallon containers of water. We keep an open one tethered to the middle step of the companionway dispensing tepid water into plastic mugs. Yuk.

6 oranges not yet rotten
1 mango
1 apple
1 avocado
2 packets of gammon steak
1 smoked sausage
2 packets of Swiss cheese (warm and smelly)
2 packets of feta cheese (ditto)
lots of pasta
lots of rice
lots of nasty tinned soup
lots of Ritz crackers

Plus Louis's personal store-cupboard of horrible but hearty ready meals in tins and packets and Oreos, flavoured with every additive in the book. This is the supply he dumped into the trolley when we were shopping at Newport with a sideways glance daring me to challenge him. It's as well he did.

Stef is very relaxed about food, and it won't hurt him to lose a few pounds, but my supplies list does nothing to reassure Louis who resembled a coat hanger when we set off and now looks like Hansel after a few weeks in the witch's cage.

And it's all my fault.

CHAPTER 35

⚓

The best swimming pool in the world

I don't know what day it is. No idea what the date is.

Midmorning, Stef starts up the engine to see how much diesel is left and asks for the twentieth time why tanks don't have marks to tell you how full/empty they are. He sets a more northerly course.

'Has Mum seen the other side of the chart?' Louis asks.

The chart has been open on the nav table since we set off, folded so that we can see the east coast of America, Bermuda and the pencil marks showing the boat's position. Since the marks have now reached the fold, I kid myself that we are nearly there. Louis opens up the chart to show me the uninterrupted acres of blue still to be crossed. I don't want to know this.

A flotilla of Man o' War, tilting in the current, float past the boat and prompt my menfolk to discuss the weapon most suited for their destruction.

Stef says, 'Hunter S. Thomson would have used a magnum as his weapon of choice.'

My husband is a mine of information. You could dig into the seams for a lifetime and still there would be facts to dredge up from the bottom of his memory. He is a facts sponge. He is filling up my son's brain, pouring the diesel of information into the tank. The men talk more facts while I worry about food and toilet rolls and mixed metaphors.

After four hours of motoring – yes, the skipper has allowed us to turn on the engine – we decide to stall the boat because we can't motor into infinity, the noise is horrible, and there may be zero wind for many more hours. Or days. Scarlet glides quietly and smoothly to a complete halt and I recite lines from Coleridge's Ancient Mariner.

There is nothing for it but to enjoy the heat and silence and go for another swim. Let me tell you that this is the best, most perfect, most satisfying swim in the world. Water like silk, sensual and tender. Bruised limbs cushioned and caressed by the ocean, soothed by stretching. I do my usual slow and effortless breaststroke, making frogs' legs before kicking away, opening my arms as wide as they can reach. We float effortlessly in tepid water, one eye open for the Portuguese. While we luxuriate in the best swimming pool in the world, Louis's voice floats across to me:

'Old fishermen tell stories about sailors who cross the ocean, then climb overboard one calm day and simply swim away, lured by mermaids or the ocean or insanity.'

I can understand that. It is so easy to swim here you feel you could drift away for miles and miles until you forget all about swimming back. A circular horizon of sea and sky, so blue you can't tell where they meet.

It is hard to get out, in every sense. Louis, tall and light, gets a foot easily on the fender and with one pull he is on deck. Stef (fourteen stone when we set off but considerably less now) clings to the fender, struggles, falls back, clings, pulls and finally gets his six foot four frame up. I can't even manage to hang on to the fender; my arms have lost all their strength. The other two could leave me here and motor off, and there would be nothing I could do. Four arms reach down and drag me up. Today – now – we are all in love with the ocean.

Stef and Louis fall asleep in the cockpit.

Later I make supper – onion, potato and cheese omelettes with hot cardboard-textured pizza base for bread. To hold the frying pan under the grill so that the cheese on top melts and bubbles and the omelette puffs up, I need to sit on the floor with the grill at eye level. I drip sweat. Not into the omelette. The result is excellent. We wash it down with warm beer.

I am aware how much I am writing about food. And thinking about it.

11p.m.

The good times didn't last.

Conditions are horrible. No wind plus huge waves 'of the wrong frequency' as Stef calls them, make Scarlet roll like a pig. A heavy hardback book flies across the cabin and thumps me on the head. The sails, mast and rigging groan and bang. I endure this for a couple of hours but it doesn't half fray the nerves, and now I'm begging Stef to take the sails down so that we can get some sleep. He does it. He's learning that the crew's fuse is shorter than when we set off.

Next day, while we photograph another sunset, a sail appears briefly on the horizon and for the first and only time on our trip, we have company. We are so excited that I get on the VHF, just to hear the voice of another human being. I am the designated radio ham, since the other two loathe phones. I must remember to observe the correct protocol and speak formally.

'This is yacht Scarlet, Scarlet, Scarlet. Calling all vessels . . .'

No reply.

'This is Scarlet, Scarlet, Scarlet . . .'

'Got any milk?' A voice calls over my shoulder into the mike. 'What about a pizza? Takeaway pizza?'

No-one answers, but I am overjoyed that we have not killed Louis's wicked sense of humour.

Over the next ten days, we glimpse only one yacht rolling about maybe five miles off, but can't raise anyone on the VHF. He probably leaves his off just as we do, and he probably hasn't seen us, just as we may well have missed boats ourselves. Our two boats pursue parallel courses, but we leave him behind in an hour.

Night watch.

The first three hours pass easily for once because I feel calm and at peace. When you are in tune with the ocean, when it's not knocking the hell out of you, it is a pleasure to lie out here under the stars being carried along gently and quietly. Louis has lent me his iPod. I make myself comfortable on cushions in the cockpit, and listen to the first chapter of the first book of Harry Potter. I vowed I would never read those damn books, and after an hour or two I decide I was right. Never mind wizards, the ocean is magical enough.

Stef joins me out here. The moon has not yet risen so there are no silvery broken mirrors on the surface of the water. The sea is dark, very, very dark. I have never seen blackness so black as this night sea. In the city there is always yellowy light after dark, and even in the country there is light somewhere in the distance. But here you can see nothing as you look over the back and sides of the boat. It is impenetrable. If you were to fall overboard you would vanish forever into a black hole.

Stef is thinking along the same lines which is hardly surprising given the all-consuming presence of the darkness. He initiates a refresher course on what to do if one of us falls in, but we disagree about the order of the three emergency procedures, and discuss which sequence would offer the best chances for the poor soul who is in the water. Our discussion focuses on the worrying fact that it will take several minutes to complete all three manoeuvres. If you go below first to press the Man Overboard button, then you have lost sight of your drowning man. If you throw the horseshoe first, you will have put enough space between you and your man overboard for the MOB to be inaccurate. We decide:

1. Throw the emergency horseshoe
2. Turn the boat around
3. Go to the nav table and press the MOB button

We look at the horseshoe on the rails and realise it has no light on it. This is really stupid. We bought a light for it, but the job of attaching it somehow got forgotten. We flash our Woolworth's torch, batteries almost flat, over the water to see how much light it gives us; about as much as a small candle. Useless! We dig into the pit of one of the lockers until we find the new search light we bought in Newport. It doesn't work.

OK, all discussion of sequence of activities is purely theoretical because it's curtains if someone falls overboard. We certainly need something more effective than a foam horseshoe without a light for the drowning and fast-vanishing person in the water. How about a string of Ikea waterproof fairy lights which would make a pretty trail in the water? Light-up antennae to wear on a headband – mandatory for anyone in the cockpit at night?

On this comforting note, I go to bed and leave Stef on watch. I hope he doesn't fall overboard.

CHAPTER 36

⚓

We make bread and hit the forties

MAYBE 27TH OR 28TH JUNE 2005

We are all a bit frustrated that we are not making more nautical miles. The wind is light and fitful so we're still wallowing about and in need of a boost. Lynn suggests fresh bread.

We have made sporadic but abortive attempts to light the oven ever since leaving Newport but while the burners on top are easy to light, the oven has defeated us. There is some safety override which we haven't found. All searches for the book of words have come to naught. Looking for the twentieth time for the safety catch, and trying all combinations of pressing relevant knobs and clicking the lighter, I hit on the solution. The button is in a daft place on top of the stove, next to the gas rings, and looks mechanical rather than electrical.

Lighting the oven turns out to be a two man job. One holds down the lighter-button on top while the other sprawls on the floor, head inside the oven, while pushing in the thermostat control and clicking the lighter. All three manoeuvres must happen simultaneously. The oven lights, and, after what seems ages, we can release the top button and it stays lit. Huge satisfaction in small achievements! Now we shall have bread!

Lynn sets to and soon the bread is rising. The oven is really hot now, and in goes the loaf. In half an hour the best bread smell ever escapes into the cockpit; it is surprising that all the fish aren't swimming round the boat in anticipation. At sea, smell is much sharper, and bread appetite stronger, and soon a bread frenzy ensues. Like a shoal of fish tearing at a floating crust, three of us dismember the loaf with bare hands. Maybe the provisions will get us to the Azores after all. Morale rockets! The oven is wonderful for a sailing boat oven, good even by home standards: heavy stainless steel American engineering, when they still made things.

The following day, with progress no better, we decide that it is time to burn some diesel. The batteries are nearly down, the wind is down, and spirits are definitely down with so much wallowing, so now is the time to use the iron tops as my father always called it. We motor for ten hours at about 5 knots. Gently does it! The revs must stay down to protect our jury-rigged alternator. We cover just fifty miles, a mere drop in the ocean, but it could save a day, or even two, getting to the wind. Frequent inspections of the alternator are positive; there's no unwarranted vibration.

We turn the engine off during dinner time and enjoy a couple of hours of peace. For a while we have 3 knots of breeze – enough to stop the wallowing – but it soon dies again.

On my watch in the early hours, there's a breath of wind. Perhaps it will prove just another zephyr blowing in circles for ten minutes but I decide it's worth unfurling the genoa. It's no good sitting about when there's wind. So it's out with the genoa on the opposite side to the main – goose winged with one sail either side of the mast – and we get a good 2 knots out of it. Goose-winged is fussy because it only permits a few degrees deviation from the course before everything collapses, but I like it. The wind vane cannot cope because the apparent wind is barely 2 knots so I turn on the electric autopilot and we glide across a moonlit sea. Magic! After the dieseling day and the wallowing night before, this is peace.

I stretch out in bliss across my usual ledge behind the wheel. I get up and root about every twenty minutes or so, and the second or third time I hear a swoosh just off the bow. A school of dolphins, about five I think, lit by the moonlight, are playing off the starboard bow. And the wind is no longer just a sequence of puffs but a steady reassuring draw giving us nearly 3 knots.

An hour later we have 6 knots of wind, and by morning when Lynn comes out on watch I can tell her that there are 7 knots of southerly wind giving us 4 knots through the water on the desired easterly course. By noon we're approaching the magic 40th parallel.

There's no white line on the ocean, but the wind fills in right on cue, so that by dinner we are heading just north of east in 15 knots of wind, making six and a half through the water with a knot of current behind us: seven and a half over the ground.

It has taken ten days or so to get 400 miles east of Newport. That's an average of 40 miles per day, gaining 2 knots on course 'as the fish swim'. We've logged more than a thousand miles through the water most of which were done in the early blow. Right royal incompetence! More haste less speed when it comes to east coast depressions and stepping onto the roundabout at the wrong point. If we'd got off from Newport into comparable south westerlies, and the wind hadn't veered NE, we'd have got to where we are now in three days instead of ten. With rather less ruffled feathers. And it would have saved two mutinies.

The roaring Forties! It's all true, even if it is just a breeze and the roaring forties are in the other hemisphere. We are finally on our way.

Chapter 37

Time

We're close reaching between 5 and 8 knots, with occasional bursts of nine. The wind direction amazes us with its constancy. It is eerie and exactly what we read about in *Ocean Passages*. We keep making minor course adjustments of a few degrees, and when we get as far as 43 degrees, we take a very definite right turn. So it is slightly baffling that our evening position plotting on the big chart comes out as an elegant arc as if some autopilot were calculating the exact great circle route.

As the first water tank runs empty with a last rusty splurge and cough, we switch to the second and last tank. We've been careful with water. We've washed up in sea water. We've cooked in half salt, half fresh. We've used minimal fresh water for ourselves, just enough to get the salt water off the skin, and clean the teeth. No clothes washing at all. But we are still using more than I calculated, unless of course the tank is leaking. With the amount of sea water in the bilge, a few gallons of fresh would not be noticeable.

On my way out to my early morning watch I note that Stef is asleep in his bunk in the company of:
  1 emergency rucksack
  1 Tupperware box of chocolate Oreos
  Louis's camera, t-shirt and shorts
  Stef's swimming trunks

1 disgusting sheet
1 disgusting blanket.

A hand reaches out and grabs me as I go past. We hope that our son remains asleep and is spared any embarrassment. The ship's clock chimes four. I love that clock, whose cheerful chimes bear no relation whatsoever to real time. Real time (is there such a thing?) is nine o'clock. It's a proper nautical clock that chimes four-hour watches, though what it chimes is anything from one to thirteen at random.

I make coffee in the pan. The cafetière was smashed to smithereens on Day Two and Louis rightly scolded me severely for having glass on board. We eat flapjack-granola out of bowls. I feel content. This day continues in its gentle, unchallenging way, a welcome relief after the madness of the initiation week. We are sailing east, making a steady 6 knots on the course we need.

In the evening we try to work out what day it is. After much finger-counting, we decide unanimously on Sunday though which Sunday no-one knows. Stef is about to put a marker on the Gecko, when he notices his watch, and remembers that his watch shows the date – one of those despised functions. Duh!!! For the past ten days he has been wearing a watch which tells us what day and date it is. And we are four days out of synch. It is not Sunday but Thursday. We are so addled that we never do work out whether this is the previous Thursday or the next Thursday, from the Sunday. Do you follow me?

What would the ancient mariner have made of our timekeeping? Before electronic position finding, exact date and time to the split second were the only way of calculating longitude. Our four days out of synch would probably have put our position somewhere in the Himalayas. Now that we have GPS and a digital calendar, my mind has rebelled by forgetting I have the date on my watch. Maybe part of wanting to get away from it all.

Now the wind is settled and constant, we barely touch the Minotaur though we admire and praise it frequently, and we do minimal sail trimming. The weather is warm and kind and we are a long way from any shipping lanes, making watches more relaxed. All told, conditions are just about perfect.

I couldn't sleep last night. My sofa ledge is too narrow for a spread-eagle sleeper like me. I may be small but I take up a lot of room in bed. I want to s . . . t . . . r . . . e . . . t . . . c . . . h out with my arms and legs flung wide. At 12.30 a.m. I got up and found Louis asleep on watch in full foul weather gear – after telling me in no uncertain terms that I had to keep scanning the horizon and watch like a hawk for container ships. Louis is doing more than his body can manage with four hour watches in the middle of the night. I sent him to bed, took over, and sat dreamily in the cockpit until 2 a.m.

When you sit in the cockpit in the dark, thoughts are random, surprising and sometimes surreal. I was thinking about instruction leaflets. This is from the one that came with our new frying pan:

'Do not operate this equipment in a room with a domesticated bird. The lungs of a domestic bird cannot cope with the fumes of a non-stick frying pan.'

No more or less bizarre than the other stuff that floats around in the small dark hours.

CHAPTER 38

An underhand change of course

When I rise, I immediately sense the tension round the boat. This is unusual because amazingly we have pulled along together very well with barely a cross word. Apart from the mutiny.

My men folk are tight-lipped and clearly angry with each other. Louis tells me that his father has taken a sneaky, unilateral decision to change course. What is more, he is swearing blind that we all agreed on it. Yet nothing has been said out loud so this is worryingly devious.

The agreement, when we turned east after being stuck in the Gulf Stream, when the chance of reaching the Chesapeake was diminishing by the day, was that we would sail for the Azores. I know that. Louis knows that. Now my husband, who can blur reality and his vivid thinking until they are indistinguishable, is talking and behaving as if the agreed plan was to head straight for the Canaries. He has thrown a switch in his own mind and assumes it has activated similar switches in ours. That's the benign interpretation. The other possibility is that he is hoping that the crew are so knocked off that they do not notice that he is manoeuvring us, whenever he can, a few degrees further south. Ah, but we do. We do.

OK, we have to have this out in the open. Louis and I challenge Stef and ask him what is going on. Stef tells us that our destination has always been the Canaries. Not quite true because while this was our original, intended destination, a lot of troubled water has passed under the bridge since then. My husband is a philosopher in his day job, and very nimble

167

with the verbal contortions, so arguing with him is like playing catch with a bar of wet soap. I speak up, pointing out that the Azores were also mentioned at that crucial decision-making moment when we were going round in circles. The Azores are right en route to the Canaries so won't mess up our journey.

Louis has played a key role in this voyage. It was he who intervened and insisted that we change course when the skipper became catatonic with anxiety and the crew were half-dead with cold and seasickness. At the nav table he has been steadily pushing us north, determined to pick up the forties, a strategy which has paid off because now we are moving at a steady 5-6 knots on exactly the course we need. And while Louis is playing by the textbook, Stef is being underhand. Whenever Louis goes off watch or is asleep, his father, under the pretext of adjusting the sails, steers us further south. Louis claims it is intentional, a ploy to move the boat so far south that we will miss the Azores altogether because if you don't approach these islands from the north, you don't reach them at all. If this is the plot, then we would be adding another thousand miles to the trip without stopping to re-provision. And we need more food.

The tension mounts. Stef and Louis argue. For a navigator to confront and disagree with a skipper is fine and kosher, but for a son to confront and disagree with his father is a different ball game altogether. The kindest interpretation of what is going on is that Stef thinks we have discussed heading straight for the Canaries, but a more realistic view is that he is trying to slip this one past us. My son is adamant that we stick to our plan to stop in the Azores to re-provision, which means a manageable two weeks more sailing. I agree with Louis. Wholeheartedly. Stef sulks. I can almost hear his brain cogs turning as he rehearses new arguments to get us back on the other course but if he tries this one again, it will be me he has to deal with. To prevent our son's health deteriorating to the point where he may be bed bound again for years, we must head for the Azores, feed him up, and put him on a plane home. He won't make it as far as the Canaries.

Apart from this very significant father-son collision, it has been a quiet day and I've slept a lot. All I've done is polish the ship's clock and the barometer. Polishing the clock has stopped its eccentric and random chiming; all we get now is one chime or none. I've made a good loaf of bread, and we have eaten pork and bean soup for supper with the last mango shared between us.

Our son is living on his reserve tank. I also sense that he is becoming bored with our company and our journey because now that our course is fair, his thoughts and conversation turn increasingly to home and his girlfriend. I have great admiration for him, living amicably alongside his mum and dad in such close quarters but, as he says in response to my acknowledgment, "It works because we have a common purpose. We are taking Scarlet to Europe."

I don't recognise any of this. My lovely wife is back in Drama School. It is true that the original plan was to go straight to the Canaries without stopping at the Azores. It is true that I was concerned about stopping in Bermuda because technically the VAT on Scarlet would become immediately payable. But it is also true that because of the behaviour of the Azores high, the best route to the Canaries passes right by the Azores. To try to cut the corner south of them is very likely to lead to being becalmed. So for whatever reason I was adjusting course on that morning, it was not to make a choice for the Canaries rather than the Azores. I was fully resigned to braving the fiscal realities for my son who is now a pressing medical problem.

Chapter 39

⚓

Internal and external geography

The crew has become very food oriented, trying to eat back the body-weight lost in the cold mist. Evening meal times are high points where Lynn works one-pot magic on the stove and food has never tasted this good. We usually eat in the cockpit, three of us lined up on the leeward bench. The rest of the day we interact in pairs since the third is usually asleep, but during evening mealtimes we all come together. We talk but, writing now, it's quite hard to remember and recreate the conversations. At sea all is here and now, regaining something of a largely lost childhood capacity for absorption in the moment. For me, the nearest land-based activity to this absorption in the sea is when the muse is dictating fluently and the pages follow one after another with complete immersion.

The homogeneity of the sea is a blue illusion put about by cartographers. Even in our ten days' thrall, with steady wind and sea, everything changes to stay the same. The light changes colour each moment, especially as the cauliflower cumulus track over us, and the sea mutates from blue to grey to green to black and back through indigo. We often see dark shreds of rain falling out of the bottom of the clouds, but in the current weather it rarely gets down to sea level, and never where we are. Out here in the deep ocean, the swell is much more regular than in coastal waters, but still there are changes to the texture as swells, generated thousands of miles away, cross cut each other, each wave a different shape. When the wind pipes up, a scattered herd of white horses progress across our close-reaching course, each looking certain to jump the cockpit rail but just as certainly tucking their heads under the stern at the last moment. Scarlet bucks and slides down their backs. Everything flows. Heraclitus must have been a sailor.

Description is a puny weakling set to the task of reproducing experience at sea. People ask what on earth we did with ourselves for all that time, but time goes quickly. The problem in the recounting is that time passes in so many different ways. The physical absorption is total but this is only part of the story because while this concentration keeps the top layer of the mind occupied, it frees the usually silent layers so that they can be heard. Faced with a total lack of landmarks by which to get its bearings, my mind conjures up a definite seascape out the mental geography I spoke out of before.

Thomas Gladwin wrote an account of the Polynesian Puluwat Islanders and their navigational feats that took them from pinprick atoll to pinprick atoll, separated by hundreds of miles of featureless water, guided only by the stars, with inevitable death the consequence of missing their targets. He describes the islanders' sea lore, the sea monsters and mermaids that populated their Pacific. Even though these journeys seem to have little more pragmatic or economic significance than do our own voyagings, nevertheless the Pulawatese spent years in navigation school learning this lore, and the master navigator was indeed exalted among islanders. Their enterprise appears to be an elaborate exercise in daring, prediction, and control of nature through knowledge. Gladwin describes the islanders' experience of their mythical creatures as real, marking real places on the sea by which they steer their passage, while we in the developed world can only understand them as a mythical menagerie.

I read Gladwin as a student and was struck by the oppositeness of Puluwat and western conceptions, but I was also left wondering whether there wasn't a more direct and truer way of reading their experience. What could they possibly mean by learning that the route from X to Y was to sail one point south of Antares to the place where the two dolphins pirouette, and then turn starboard two points as far as the blue mermaid? Sailing east on the 40th parallel, I begin to have some inkling of the experience they report. For them, the system of sea marks is a socialised system, related to the memorisation of the astronomical and other navigational data which they can't look up in the Almanac they don't carry. For me this experience of steering to definite places, alongside highways in my imaginary geography, is an individual narrative welling up from some deep recess of my mind, and released because the chattering layers are anaesthetised. Perhaps this is not some elaborate metaphor after all but something really experienced. Obviously the dolphins don't pirouette, and the mermaid, while perhaps a vivid blue, is not sitting on the sea. I'm not that daft. No, these are the landmarks of an inner landscape and perhaps most easily thought of as mnemonics – aids to memory.

The Pulueatese learnt their system of seamarks somewhat as Cicero's rhetoric students learnt to place their mnemonic notes for their speeches in places within buildings. When it came to giving the speech, the orator took an imaginary tour of the building and recovered the topoi (topics) of the speech from the places where he had lodged them while composing. An orator used the same building each time he composed a new speech. If you had to learn your navigation tables by heart, the occasional blue mermaid might make them vivid just as Cicero instructs.

The reason Gladwin's account fascinated me as a student was very personal. I had, and still have, the experience of an idiosyncratic mnemonic place system. It is idiosyncratic twice over. Straightforwardly, it is my own system of places. It seems to function as something of the inverse of Cicero's well known system, and I have not been able to find any others who report the same experience. My system is not something deliberately done to remember things but rather something I have noticed that my memory does of its own accord. Rather than consciously placing things to be remembered in places that I know, and then deliberately retrieving them by mental travel, I am aware of being *in* a certain place as I think about specific, usually rather abstract, ideas. These associations of places and ideas are persistent and consistent over many years. I still experience being in the same places when I return to ideas I first met as a student forty years ago. These places that ideas stick themselves on are never consciously chosen, and are still emerging in my mental life, usually when I am trying to learn something new and difficult.

The reader may or may not be interested to know that this particular part of the voyage has, as I write, become linked with a place a few hundred yards from the house where I grew up. A few yards down the lane from our house, outside a rundown farmyard was an ancient rickety wooden stand on which the farmer stood his churns of milk so that the collector could roll them on to his lorry and take them off to the dairy. I am positioned by that old oak stand as I think back over this section of our voyage. This place belongs to an older part of my real childhood's mental geography but has now formed a connection with this part of the Atlantic and, as I write, comes back to mind. All these mental geographies are part of the inner structure of my mental life. They are far too systematic and long lasting, and engender emotions that are far too powerful, to be merely happenstantial. They are, like all inner structures, accessible only indirectly. When I am thinking about a particular idea, I have the simultaneous and intense experience of being in a very definite place. Those places are where I am while I sit here at my desk, or in Scarlet's cockpit, thinking and feeling certain thoughts.

Sailing out into the Atlantic seems to have cleared away the mental litter that blows around the civilised mind and has made more vivid my underlying mental geographies. One night I am travelling to Texas and the next sitting by the milk churns on their stand down by the farmhouse.

What I do not do out here sailing is spend much time thinking purposefully about all those things which at home one wishes one had time to think about purposefully. Out here, thoughts are even more their own mistresses who appear at their own whim and, just as capriciously, make their own curtain calls. But then, it has always been obvious to me that thoughts entertain thinkers, rather than the other way about. Nobody is more thoroughly gripped than a person with an octopus of an idea.

The boundary between wake and sleep is different at sea, in line with the total physical absorption in the sailing. Five minutes in a bunk and I am away with the fishes, deep asleep and dreaming. But this dreaming is a continuation of waking. It is embedded in the physicality of a boat in sea. The slightest shift in the wind direction or a slight change in wind strength or wave pattern, and I am awake, yet barely experience waking up. The most vivid example was crossing into the Gulf Stream asleep while Louis was helming, but that is only one example with an easily given reference. Even while I slept, I experienced that journey as clearly as if I had been awake. It was a voyage of vivid but ineffable experiences.

CHAPTER 40

⚓

You can't photograph the ocean

EARLY JULY 2005

Despite my last ditch attempts in Newport to get a memory card for Louis's camera, what I bought still won't connect. This means that he's limited to about fifty pictures for the whole trip which imposes interesting and instructive editorial decisions. It's surprisingly hard to render our voyage in images. It would be easier to hover outside the boat and photograph inwards rather than facing out on to the great expanse – an analogy for writing about inner and outer spaces perhaps. Dropping the camera man off in the dinghy in anything other than flat calm is not this skipper's idea of responsibility. Recovering a cameramen from the dinghy would be easy enough in flat calm, but then pictures of a becalmed and rolling boat are not what we're after. And since we are doing nearly 8 knots, getting the paparazzi back on board would not be easy. The action photos will have to wait for inshore days.

Looking outwards, the most obviously photogenic events are the sunsets, lurid reds and greens sometimes spread around three quarters of the horizon. There is one memorable evening when great black tufts of stuff hang in a bruised sky, like the cataracts in moss agate, or perhaps some deity's eyebrows. These displays compel moods. The idea that they are just some random physical phenomenon is implausible in the extreme. The sky glowers down sending shivers through the body into the pit of the stomach, or emotions soar to the sublime, well beyond prose's capacity for purple.

A library of sunsets rapidly accumulates. Editorial meetings to make space on the camera are fascinating. Evenings are spent making a selection as the camera is passed around and images are viewed on the little back screen. It becomes an after-dinner ritual. Long after we're back on land, the pictures of the sunsets can still conjure up the original evenings, and each really is a particular evening. Nature considers repetition beneath her.

After evenings come nights, warm and welcoming and sprinkled with stars. As we lie on deck, Louis announces shooting stars and teaches Lynn the technique of attending through the corner of one's eye. Once you get the knack, the sky is riven with shooters, mostly just short hyphens, but occasionally a full line blazed down the page.

Saturday 2nd July
(I'm guessing. I haven't a clue what the date is).

On this, our first voyage, we have been drip-fed magic moments. Here comes another. We are cruising along at 8 knots with Scarlet beautifully balanced, putting her shoulder in. We have a soldier's wind, stable and easy. Louis and I jump up into the dip in the mainsail, just above the boom, and sit with our backs against the sail and our faces in the sun.

Later I dig out the very last lump of rancid butter, kept back from the cauldron of flapjack (just in case, just in case what?) and make a cake. No scales, no measures, no cake tin. I use brown sugar, honey, white flour, slivered almonds and three precious eggs which are not blue. This random concoction, poured into the bread tin, produces a very moist, very buttery cake with a big dent in the middle.

The good wind lasts all day and into the night, giving us a much needed break. Supper is pasta, smoked sausage and cheese (again) and an apple between the three of us. Again I am harking on about food, something which, in normal circumstances, I'm not all that interested in.

I am on watch until 1.30 a.m. with Scarlet still racing along at 6–7 knots. We are on the tack that tips me out off my narrow ledge onto the floor, so when Stef wakes and takes over, I wriggle into his bunk and pass out. But then he is back, too tired tonight to do his watch. I bed down on the settee that took the soaking, but sleep eludes me there.

The dank, salty smell and the feel of wet sofa fabric on my bare skin depresses me so I go back on deck again. It is 4 a.m. and Scarlet is still going strong.

1290 nautical miles to go to reach the Azores.

*

We are about two-thirds of the way to the Azores from our point of decision. The sky begins to descend. The wind picks up slightly and slowly the seas build. Lynn uses the VHF to hail a tanker passing on the horizon and asks for a weather forecast. The navigator is extremely helpful. He goes off air for fifteen minutes and comes back with a thorough search of all the low pressure activity from Florida to the Canaries. There are a couple of shallow lows, one centered about three hundred miles astern and tracking to pass well north of us. This is the only one that could affect us. We later speak to a couple of other ships before we get home. The navigators, without exception, go out of their way to help us. There really does seem to be some brotherhood of the sea. Even if they are ploughing by in something the size and shape of an office block, with more weather information than the Met Office had available thirty years ago, they seem genuinely interested in what we amateur idiots are up to, and are understanding when we so incompetently try to imitate their skills.

A day later, and the sky continues to lower its lid. The wind is up from 17 to about 25 knots and the sea has built up big and grey. We're sailing across a big swell which must be coming from the depression tracking north of us, feeling the usual incredulity that the boat will lift itself over each peak after emerging from the trough. However many times it happens, each up and over seems a revelation. There are some dense-looking rain squalls around with slate grey wisps dropping out below them, though the first ones miss us. The combined effect of sea and sky makes for a sense of foreboding. It's not that we're worried, just that the weather directly registers its mood. This close to the elements, our mood is the sea's mood. The elements aren't angry with us. We don't have that significance.

My mood is not exactly bright when I wake. I desperately, yearningly want my own bed. I want a comfortable clean bed where I can stretch my arms and legs wide and where the sheet does not stick to me, and there isn't a steel band playing its metallic tunes under my bed in the water tank.

My guilt is getting to me more and more because Louis is not getting nearly enough to eat and there is not much I can do about it. We eat buttery cake for breakfast. The other two are in better shape today while I am puffy-eyed and stupid. On we go at a steady 6.5 knots, not as fast as yesterday, but fast enough, and in the right direction.

My husband chooses today to express his upset that I still call everything by the wrong name. In my personal nautical dictionary fenders are called bollards, sheets are called red, blue or spotted ropes, the horrible lee cloth which I tried one night with disastrous results, is a loin cloth. And so on. I'm a word-monger and quite like coining my own terms, but, my husband points out, this is not the place to do it. It is dangerous to shout out the wrong name – and I have to agree. So up we go on deck for a strict lesson during which I must concentrate and be serious. I name the halyards and sheets, distinguish between standing and running back stays, learn which rope is attached to what. I knew it all so well on our old boat-share boat, but this one is rigged quite differently and I have to start all over again. Because I do not intuitively understand how a boat functions or how it sails, because I have no conceptual grasp of the principles, everything has to be done with labels and signposts.

I'm going below now to wipe the sticky horizontal and vertical surfaces. I can do that.

Oh no! OH NO! The boat is filling up with sea water again so that to get from A to B below, we have to paddle through a shallow lake. My hands feel sticky, my face feels sticky, everything is sticky.

As the afternoon wears on, the wind slowly gets up and the sea grows bigger and bigger until the waves are topped with white horses. I am still mopping up water on my hands and knees, squeezing a sponge into a bucket, when I am thrown from one side of the saloon to the other, bucket upturned on the floor. I scramble back up and cling to the work-surface but another wave sends me bouncing round the galley into all the sharp handles and hinges and sticking out bits of metal that the idiot designers put there. Finally I am sliding on my bum towards the cupboards opposite the galley and come to rest pressed hard against the louvered doors. The next time I struggle out of my clothes, I count twenty-seven bruises on one leg.

By early evening the wind is blowing 20-25 knots, nothing alarming, just very uncomfortable in these huge seas. Scarlet wallows and slews while maintaining a hell of a speed. She is well heeled over as we surf down the ski-slope waves. I wedge myself with my back against the cupboard and my feet against the cooker, the only possible position for cooking supper. The worst bit is getting from this secure position to the sink because my grabbing hands are occupied with transferring a large pan of almost boiling water and cooked pasta to the sink to be drained in a sieve. I need to make this move without pouring the contents of the pan all over myself, and without being jettisoned across the saloon with it still in my hands. Phew – that done and the pasta safely in the sieve – I return to my wedged spot to fry smoked sausage, tinned mushrooms, and to throw in a tin of tomatoes grabbed, in another minute's lull, from the cupboard over the settee. This mixture simmers while I draw breath. With a quick crab-wise movement to the sink and back to the cooker, I grab the sieve and add the pasta to the pan. Stir. I open up the fridge lid. It slams back down on my hand because there is no way of hooking it open. I have to dive down into the black hole balanced on one leg, holding the lid up with one hand so it does not fall and trap the other one. I retrieve the smelly, warm cheese and squash it through the holes of the grater into the pot. Stir again. I'm streaming with sweat but safely braced hard against my back support. Now I must time my exit carefully. I wait for a moment's lull, then yell, 'Dinner is on its way' while I make a bolt for the companionway, banging my elbows as I go. Stef grabs the hot pan from me. I climb out. Sit down. Spoon portions into three bowls.

Wedged on the floor, our backs to the lockers, we try to get food into our mouths as the waves tower first on one side up to the gunnels then the other. If you time each spoonful with our exact position through the waves, you can sometimes hit the target of your mouth. The rest goes everywhere. We are too tense now to enjoy the meal but it's fuel. Only Louis manages a second helping.

After supper Louis tries to photograph the waves, to capture just how enormous they are, swirling all around the boat, but after many attempts, he looks at his digital images and says, 'They look like we're on a calm sea off Brighton.'

CHAPTER 41

The undoing of Louis

Scarlet is roaring along in a somewhat alarming fashion. Fast is good but this is out of control. The wind registers 25 knots. Our speed over the ground is 11 knots then 12 knots. There is nothing for it but to reef the mainsail and somehow reduce the size of the genoa. While the first task is possible, the second is not. We have no self-furling mechanism because the rope broke some time ago. It's a terrifying prospect because the genoa is one vast sail with a hell of a force in her. In this weather, in these seas, no-one can man handle it.

Wearing safety harnesses, Louis and I put a reef in the mainsail, then another, and are rewarded by our skipper with top marks for speed and coordination. But who is going to risk life and limb up in the bows to roll the genoa by hand? Scarlet is pitching in huge seas with waves breaking every few seconds over the bows and coach roof. Whoever goes up will be instantly soaked and will have a hard time staying upright and on board, let alone trying to hand-roll a massive sail with an unimaginable force in it.

Stef strips off to his trunks, puts on a harness and crawls along the deck while Louis takes the helm and I pay out and pull back the gib sheets to try to hold the sail steady. We can see Stef trying to turn the roller and we can also see that the sail is not winding up. He sits there in the bows turning and turning while the waves crash over him until he is beaten and crawls back. He says, 'The wheel goes round but the sail doesn't furl.' Louis offers to go and look.

I know that Louis is not physically fit for this Herculean task. He should not do it. Like his father, he strips down to his boxer shorts, puts on a harness and crawls out along the deck, ducking the bucket loads of sea water which hit him slap in the face. I am tense and taut with fear as wave after wave come down on top of him. Now we watch him in the bows, watch him get the sail in and round the roller for a few turns, and watch it slip out again. Back he comes.

'I need something to use as a handle,' he says between chattering teeth.

His skin is all goose bumps and he is shivering violently. I pass him the bilge pump handle and back he goes. His lean, almost naked figure rises up with each wave and crashes down again. How can he keep two hands on the winding device and one hand on the boat to stop himself being thrown across it, or overboard? It is agony watching him because I know how cold he is and how much this is taking out of him.

Back he comes a second time, soaked and shaking, white as a ghost.

'Lost the pump handle overboard,' he manages to say. His mouth is too numb to speak.

What to use to reduce the sail for almost an hour in treacherous conditions? The light is fading fast. We have to find a way of getting the sail furled before dark when it will be too dangerous even to try. It is 8 p.m. The men have been trying to reduce the sail for almost an hour. My mind has gone blank and Stef is silent. Louis comes to the rescue again.

'Broom handle,' he says.

He is too cold and exhausted to say more than one or two words at a time. We dig in the locker for the broom and search for a saw to cut it down to size but find the saw has lost its blade. One revenge after you have invested too much effort, and we are too tired to think clearly. Louis props the broom between port and starboard lockers and jumps on it.

I go up on the foredeck while Louis eases the genoa sheet from the cockpit to take off some of the tension. We still have no furling line. I can't turn the drum by hand at all. I come back aft and am just considering whether to bring the boat round a bit more into wind – an exciting option in these conditions – or to find something to give me some leverage, when Louis pushes past me, dives into the cockpit locker, pulls out a broom handle, jumps on it, snapping it in two, and rushes forwards, clipping his harness onto the

SHOOTING STARS ARE THE FLYING FISH OF THE NIGHT

jack-lines. He inserts the broom handle through the drum housing and turns and turns.

His father is too slow.

Heaven only knows what it takes to crawl back to the prow a third time. The boat is so unstable now with the deranged, disturbed sea and the out-of-control, crazy gib that it would only take one freak wave to knock him overboard. I don't know how he hangs on and keeps his balance in the bows while being buffeted by so much water. I know this is an ordeal for him. It is a mother's nightmare, her child at the mercy of such a terrifying sea. Stef is still silent and I sense he feels he should be doing this, not his son. We can see that Louis has managed to push the broom handle through the base of the self-furling gear and is winding. And winding. The gib gets smaller until it is a big triangle. Then a small triangle. And then a little hanky. And then nothing. Louis secures the broom handle with rope and crawls back. He is icy cold, ashen, and clearly shaken.

The foredeck is a scary spot to be. We are close to surfing down the waves in a squall beneath the overtaking cloud, and the bow is burying itself deep in each wave with oodles of sea sloshing across the foredeck. Louis struggles to tame the genoa using his improvised broom handle capstan to roll it up, while I minimise the tension by playing the genoa sheet. It takes what seems forever. Louis comes back to the cockpit having hand-furled the genoa down to a pocket handkerchief. He is sea-coloured. An able-bodied sailor would be done in after what he has just done and he is far from able-bodied. I blame myself.

I push my shaking son into the head, put the water pump on – something we no longer do – and order him to have a proper warm shower for as long as he needs to get warm, and then to get into bed. It is dark. Scarlet is making her way more calmly now. Stef and I are very subdued. There are more dangerous situations than this one, but it has been testing enough. Stef is exhausted and I am shaking so much, even though I have done nothing, that I go and lie on the settee. For a while Scarlet is left to her own devices.

At 10 p.m. Stef and Louis get up. I wonder how my husband feels about his son achieving what he himself could not manage. In all our years of sailing as a family, it has always been Stef who has taken on the most dangerous tasks or anything that required brute force and massive strength. I remember the times in the past when he has dived under the boat to free an anchor, surfacing with blood streaming from his nostrils, or when he has stood on deck in appalling conditions to untangle something that has jammed.

'That was brilliant,' he says now to his son.

Louis, always tuned in to the feelings of others, just jokes about the gib being easier to release than wind up.

'You're stronger than me,' Stef adds.

'I'm not so sure about that,' my son replies tactfully.

My husband seems to be passing the baton to the younger generation. My Herculean husband. We are all done in, physically and emotionally.

I think that Stef watches for most of the night, perhaps in recompense. I try to sleep on my ledge but muscles have to work overtime to keep me from falling on to the floor. I wedge myself into the space with every available cushion but to no avail. We are pitching. We are seesawing along. At 5 a.m. I wake Louis and ask him to swap bunks. Bless him, he offers not a word of complaint. The forward cabin bunk is wide enough for me to stretch out, and with a padding of cushions and pillows on either side, I am braced no matter what the boat does. I sleep until midday.

'We've done 142 miles in the night,' Louis tells me when I finally surface. As I take over, Stef crashes out. Louis lies down in the cockpit, looking awful. I sail Scarlet for four hours, pleased that at least I can do this, but feeling humbled by Louis's determination, when we were in trouble last night, to do whatever was necessary to make the boat safe, even to the detriment of his own health and well being. What the father was unable to accomplish, the son achieved.

With my years of experience with an illness which takes its revenge after you have made too much of an effort, I know beyond doubt that my son has pushed himself too far and will suffer the consequences. There is no road back to recovery. Anxiety keeps me company as we cruise through the waves.

Now Scarlet is reefed down to a controllable rig, still averaging 8 and a half knots in the 25 knots of wind, but, as always, happy with it, she reassures her crew.

One watch later, the wind is back to its constant 15 knots and its direction doesn't deviate more than perhaps 10 degrees during the whole frontal passage. With hindsight, we would probably have got away with not reefing, but it would have been unseamanlike in the extreme. If it weren't for Louis's shade of green when he came back from the foredeck I wouldn't give it another thought, but it takes Louis several days flat out on his bunk to begin to be able to function at all. I am kicking myself.

We sail on along the same elegant arc. There's not quite so much sun as before, though the foreboding grey has relented. We cross the shipping lane from Gran Abaco Island off the Bahamas to Gibraltar when we are about 2 degrees north of the Azores. A procession of curious metal boxes pretending to be ships churn past as if running on rails. One looks like a dry dock which is maybe what it is, and the rest are the usual office blocks. We have been gradually adjusting our course to come down from 43 north, to cross the 40th parallel at about 33 degrees west, heeding dire warnings from *Ocean Passages* about cutting the corner south too early and becoming becalmed.

Maybe Wednesday 6th July

There are a few days missing here because I've been too miserable to write. I want to get off the boat. More urgently and passionately, I want Louis to get off the boat. Guilt sits right on my shoulder, a gremlin that chides and chatters, because we have asked far too much of our son. I am beyond distress because I know from bitter experience that he has crossed the point of no return where his energy loss goes into free fall. Like a man who has jumped from a plane without a parachute, he will hit rock bottom.

Inevitably, Louis's ME symptoms return with a vengeance after his heroic gib-coiling act in the bows. He lies motionless and curled up in the captain's bunk with cold sweats, shivering, stomach cramps and muscle pain. He can't eat, not because of seasickness, but because not being able to eat without pain is part of his illness. He feels defeated and disappointed – mostly with himself and his wretched heart-sink health.

'I really thought I could do it,' he says. 'I thought I'd manage...'

'I know. But it's been much more gruelling than we imagined. You have been valiant,' I say in a vain attempt to console him.

CHAPTER 42

⚓

Whale!

Yesterday we had some surprise visits.

I was lying face down on my bunk, fast asleep, when someone pulled my legs, and a voice said, 'Quick, Mum, dolphins!' It's worth being woken up to see dolphins. We leaned over the railings and there they were, very close to the boat, arching in and out of the water. Most were small so we decided they were a family. Lovely, shimmering, playful creatures.

One morning Louis is on watch. Despite being ill he is still doing some daylight watches. We hear a yell from the cockpit.

'A whale! Get up here quick!' he bellows.

Louis doesn't do bellowing so we hit the companionway fast.

'There's a whale!' He shouts. "A whale!"

I stagger on deck in time to see an enormous brown creature as long as Scarlet making straight at our bows. The movement looks forthright, but not all out aggressive. It feels as if we're being told firmly to get off his patch. He definitely feels like a he. Either that or plain curiosity. Or just an itch he wants to scratch? Then we see a second, smaller whale further off so perhaps he is indulging in some macho whale behaviour. The huge bulky creature crossing our path swerves just as it reaches the bow. Louis drags the helm over. I can see our grey anti-fouling in a stripe on the whale's brown back where our bow has scraped a swirling pool of brown slimy water off his smooth skin. The impact is gentle, a hardly perceptible nudge. How can that many tons of whale calculate a nudge on a 12 ton boat bouncing up and down in a seaway? Louis says it was all down to the helmsman's timely action and that it would have rammed us hard and done itself some damage if the helmsman hadn't been a genius.

'I saw his eyes,' Louis says.

The whale is enormous, I'd guess forty feet, and not slender. It's easy to give a good estimation because he was briefly almost lined up alongside, just a bit shorter than our 46 feet. And then he sounds, and he's gone. We feel deserted. 'Oh please don't go, we love you so!'

The whale surfaces about fifty yards off the port bow and blows spray way up in the air. He's watching us, one eye just above his waterline. There is a second whale further out, perhaps his mate. We are all worried that we have hurt him, maybe grazed his skin. No-one seems worried that he might have hurt the boat, or us.

Thinking it over, the grey anti-fouled bottom of our boat must look somewhat whale-like, at least more like a whale than anything else in these parts. And it dawns on me that our wing keel is a dead ringer for a whale's tail. We conclude that we sailed too close to his lady love, and got the brush off. Perhaps.

Later, back home on dry land, we try to identify what sort of whale he was by looking at a whale chart in a café in Tenerife, though none of the options looks quite right. The only brown one is a Northern Bottlenose Whale which is only occasionally found where we were sailing. But maybe color isn't reliable. An adult sperm whale is too big but an immature one seems a possibility, since they seem to live almost everywhere, and especially around the Azores. Sperm whales are famously curious about boats so maybe he was just trying to play with us.

Many months later, at a conference, I meet a whale expert who asks me where we were and tells me immediately that it was a small sperm whale. Small! Meeting a big one would indeed be interesting.

A few hours later, on deck alone, I saw more dolphins, big ones this time. Three magic meetings in the space of a single day. The creatures had come to offer their greetings and consolations. They had arrived to cheer us because they sensed we were all struggling with difficult emotions. Yes, of course that's fanciful, but why not?

The night before the visitations, the wind had got up until we were way over-canvassed and the cupboards started emptying themselves again. Unbearable, this, so Stef and I went up to put a reef in the mainsail. If only wind were a bit more predictable; no sooner had we got the reef in than the wind dropped and Scarlet started to wallow from side to side. OK, back up we go. Shake out the reef. Why do these fickle wind changes always happen at night, in pitch darkness, with no moon to shine its eerie light on deck? Earlier in the trip I had poured orange juice all over my sailing gloves, making them unusable so now I am wearing the very latest in fashionable sailing gear: calamine-pink waterproof jacket, blue waterproof trousers and yellow rubber gloves. Stef pokes his salty arms down the sleeves of his heavy weather jacket but remains naked from the waist down.

Just to finish off the scene, the rain comes down, bringing angry, black seas. The clouds lower themselves to just above the boat and hover there.

I take stock below. We have one soaking wet settee covered in black hefty bags, one damp settee that wets your knickers when you sit on it, and two damp bunks. The engine is still not charging despite Stef's best efforts so we are now without lights and music. We dare not turn on the engine because we may still need what little charge is left.

I note Stef and Louis have given up washing. Louis has a dark pirate beard and hair as choppy as the ocean; Stef has grey stubble because he still shaves now and again. They lie on their sticky bunks partially or fully clothed. We have three rather nasty sheets between us. There is a single orange in the fruit crate. We have grown silent.

Padded all around with cushions I manage to lie flat without levitating every few minutes or being rolled up against the ceiling. I think of whales, imagining our visitor returning to take his revenge, swimming silently under our boat until he can lift us right out of the water. I can't sleep. I must sleep. Louis is out of action now. Stef needs me alert and able to concentrate.

The crew is down to one able-bodied adult and one who is just about surviving.

CHAPTER 43

Towards land

7TH JULY 2005

We're getting close to our first destination. Over the first twenty-four hours after we had reached the magic 40th parallel, we made over a hundred miles. Then 120, then 140. Our best day was 197 miles, with the big 200 just eluding us, even with a knot of tail-current pushing us. From there on, our plot on the chart was a beautiful arc descending across the 43rd parallel toward the Azores. The last 1500 miles have taken ten days.

Someone set the cursor on our landfall several days ago and has been reading off the miles-to-go and noting them on the log. I feel so much in the groove I could just keep going. But Louis is still struggling after his cold water treatment and thinks he's going to have to abandon ship for plane on the Azores.

Late last night, when I was on watch, the GPS unveiled a wonderful surprise. A gift. Unlike Louis, who can operate things technical without consulting the manual (bad idea, he says), I am a hopeless case. Here's what happened.

It is midnight and I have been on watch for a couple of hours while my men folk are crashed out in the Captain's bunk. I am getting bored and twitchy. I am watching the dials, watching the sails, watching the horizon and then I start to fiddle with the GPS buttons. Louis has marked the nearest island in the Azores which at this moment is 450 nautical miles away. I zoom in on the Azores, zoom out, zoom in (it passes the time) but then I notice a little piece of orange in the bare blue sea. What's that? It must be a big rock. A big rock not much smaller than the next island seems unlikely. I don't trust my brain at this time of night but even so my heart gives a little jolt as I consult the paper chart. It's not a rock, it is an island, so small that it has gone unnoticed in Louis's chart plotting. It is Flores, and it is a hundred miles nearer than our previously pinpointed destination.

Yeeha!

Whoopee!

We are one whole day closer to dry land than previous calculations had determined. I wake Stef later to tell him I'm going off duty and to give him my news, terrified that somehow I have got it wrong.

'Flores', he says, half asleep. 'Yeah! That's where we're going.'

I climb into my damp bed a whole lot happier.

When I wake, it's not raining. Cloudy, but no rain yet. Scarlet is progressing at a steady 7 knots in the right direction. I tell Louis, still in bed, about Flores, our hidden island. He gives me the thumbs up, too tired for conversation. I bake bread. Stef makes onion soup. It's just another grey day at sea.

To pass the time I list all the positive aspects of this adventure and weigh them against the negatives – as of this moment. What am I missing most? What is fulfilling? This list would of course be different on another day, at another hour, depending on sea-state, the wind, Louis's state of health, and my mood. This is today's reckoning.

The down side:

A leaking, sodden boat. In my book, this has been worse than anything, apart from Louis being so ill, but that's of another order of magnitude.

A wet bed. Same as above but more specific.

Filthy sheets. Being female, there's a limit to how much dirt, oil, sea-water, sweat and biscuit crumbs I can tolerate next to my skin. I don't think this bothers the men one bit.

No juice on waking. I just love my glass of ice-cold grapefruit juice first thing in the morning.

No yoghurt. At home I live on the stuff.

Tepid drinking water. Warm beer. I like my food and drink piping hot or icy cold.

No fruit. I exaggerate; one orange left.

Sticky skin. My ration of water does not shift the layer of salt. I want a power-shower.

Night watches. At the beginning of this voyage, we were so diligent, sticking out the full four hours while remaining alert and careful. Then we slowly reverted to mostly awake during the light, and fitfully asleep after dark. I confess there have been a few nights recently when all three of us were asleep below.

Smoked sausage, stinky cheese, pasta and tin soup. After several weeks I long for a green salad followed by a fruit salad. I am The Hungry Caterpillar.

The up side:

Scarlet. Scarlet, and Scarlet again. Our very own beautiful boat except, sod it, she leaks, her engine is tied up with string, there is no fridge, the furling gear is broken and we can't put the lights on. I may have put this in the wrong list.

We three – mother, father, son – have been confined to a boat that leaks and has an engine tied up with . . . (see above) and still we have had barely a cross word. We have worked well as a team, been supportive, been tuned in to one another's needs. I feel nothing but respect for my two men.

360 degree sunsets. A different picture postcard every evening (except when it rains or is blowing a gale).

The company of a whale, dolphins, flying fish and turtles.

Finding, settling to and enjoying a simple, basic way of living with very few complaints from any of us, however fed up we may occasionally feel.

The good communication between my husband and son as they chat all the time about boats, weather, wind, and technicalities beyond my comprehension.

We had long ago given up trying to tune in to the BBC World Service because all we managed to get was white noise. It didn't bother us at all to be out of contact because we wanted to be cast off, literally, from everyday life.

The day progresses, and then at 5 p.m., I have a strong need to hear a news bulletin. This is the first time during the trip that I have felt this need and it is quite urgent. In retrospect, I do not understand what happened here. Coincidence? Sixth sense? Why this particular moment? Look at the date. Of course it meant nothing then but this date is etched on most people's memories now. It's one of those questions: Where were you when you heard the news on 07/07? We were on a boat crossing the Atlantic. We tuned in to the news for the first time during that crossing.

I ask Louis to try to find a signal. He clips the aerial to the metal tube of our wind vane, tunes in (something he has done many times before) and immediately we hear the news of the London terrorist bombings. We are stunned. After no news for several weeks, and not wanting news, we hear loud and clear that London tube trains and a bus have been blown up. Thirty-seven dead. Seven hundred injured. Our thoughts turn to those we know who travel regularly by public transport in London. Is my other son OK? My sister? It shocks us because of the contrast between the way we are living now, in the middle of the Atlantic, alone, in complete freedom, and the way those commuters going about their ordinary and extraordinary every day lives were confronted with this.

A small sailing boat has kept us safe through violent seas, scary winds, currents. Two tube trains and a bus have been blown apart by terrorist bombs. People's lives have been changed forever.

Too awful to contemplate. Too dreadful to discuss. That evening, we sail on in silence towards the Azores, each lost in thought. I think about our freedom and security here on the ocean compared to the abrupt, cruel pain, injury and loss of life inflicted on London commuters who were unlucky enough to be going about their daily lives on the wrong day at the wrong time.

Tomorrow we should reach the Azores. Louis is now so ill that we have to get him on a plane back to Edinburgh.

PART THREE

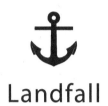

Landfall

CHAPTER 44

Flores

JULY 8TH 2005

In the small hours, as Lynn takes over the watch from me, we can make out a faint glow of light coming from Flores. By some trick of optics and meteorology, the light disappears for several hours before reappearing only after we've halved the remaining distance. Our watches are rather thorough by recent standards since we expect fishing traffic and maybe ferries, and sure enough there are quite a few lights doing nothing very interpretable, almost certainly small fishing boats.

When dawn eventually breaks, the lighthouse light is clear, and Lynn wakes me and Louis to witness landfall. It arrives right on cue.

Saturday 9th July

Last night I volunteered for the dawn watch with obvious ulterior motives. I am on deck at 4 a.m. and almost immediately see land – well, I see a misty bump in the far distance rising out of a hazy sea. Sunrise is gentle and water-washed this morning, the sea calm, the winds soft. After 2,500 nautical miles and three weeks it is difficult to grasp the fact that the shape ahead is an island. I call to Louis to come up on deck. Then Stef joins us. They assure me it will be a long time before we reach Flores, if it is Flores, and sensibly go back to bed. I stay out watching the island oh so slowly getting a little bit bigger and a bit bigger until I think I can see marks and lines on its mountain slopes. I stare at the shape for four hours in a dream but we are not much nearer.

I turn in for some sleep, having put the eBay GPS card in the old chart-plotter, and satisfied myself that the harbour at Lajes is where it should be. It is a straightforward approach with no hazards. By the time I've had a nap, we're close enough to land to see the few settlements on the west coast and the intense soft green of the mountainous island. And to smell its landy smell.

It turns out that we have not read the chart very accurately. If we had eased off a bit, we would have sailed straight into Lajes and saved ourselves some time, but as it is we are doing the scenic route, right down the West side to the southern tip. I am a bit impatient, but the others shrug their shoulders. What's a few hours in a trip of 2,500 miles?

I was expecting a bit more jubilation but Stef, far from rejoicing, is worrying out loud about the unpaid VAT on Scarlet. The reason we decided on our original plan to make landfall in the Canaries was that we would not have to pay VAT there. Stef grumbles on about the need to drop anchor, shove Louis on a plane home, and race off again. He wants us to behave like pirates. I do wish he would relax. This should be such a significant moment, but here he is making contingency plans for our escape before we have even put foot ashore after our weeks on the ocean. His disappointment at not making the Canaries direct seems to be translated into an angry worrying about VAT.

Please, just savour this moment. We are almost there.

I seem to have a problem with the timing of the expression of my emotions. They are not synchronised with others even if we are sharing, and feeling, the same experience. This is difficult for all concerned and one outcome may be that I don't often show very much emotion because the chances are I would display it at an inappropriate moment, or when no-one is around. We've had so much illness in our family – so many years upon years of chronic, life-changing illness – that the bit of my brain which deals with illness news is truly burnt out. This inability to deal with illness has somehow become crosscut with any good news that does come in.

Let me give you an example. We spot the loom of the Flores light, and know that within twelve hours we will have made it safely into harbour. At this moment, I'm on watch alone, and I don't suppose that anyone who happened to be spying on the cockpit would be able to observe the slightest hint of what I feel. Not even my wife. Maybe I'm stiller than usual while it lasts? But it is extraordinarily vivid. Something I will never forget.

As we reach the tip of the island, I get on the VHS and ask for permission to enter the marina.

'Ees not a marina,' says a welcoming Portuguese voice. 'Anchor in the bay. Have a nice stay.'

And there it is. The little bay of Flores, a safe basin surrounded on three sides by a man-made breakwater and the docks, the small village built high up the hill, and wooded cliffs falling down to the sea. On shore everything looks undeveloped, basic, and wonderfully untidy. On the seaward side, the breakwater is a mass of immense three-legged, precast blocks of concrete that look like leftover plumbing. The few straggling houses sit on top of a steep path above a traditional black and white wall. Below the cliffs on the other side of the harbour are rocks and a bit of a beach.

And then, as we round the corner, we see that all the boats anchored in the bay are of the travelling kind. You can recognise them from the wind vanes, solar panels, and washing on the rails – and all the folk on deck wave in welcome as we search for a space where we can drop anchor. We are used to bays in Greece and Croatia where most of the boats are charter boats, plastic fantastics and gin palaces crewed by couples in townie-clean shorts and t-shirts. But here are the real sailors. We feel relaxed and at home, among fellow travellers.

There's a great sense of pride in having got here. Scarlet feels like ours now and I think she is pleased with her new owners, relieved to have been set free on the ocean. We see a beach or two and the odd hut, but only a couple of villages on the whole of this coast. It looks welcoming; about the population density we feel able to deal with. 'Anyone for carrying straight on to the Canaries?' I ask.

We pull out the improvised hawsepipe plug, shackle the anchor back onto the chain, and drop it onto the rocky bottom. Holding looks dire so let's hope the weather stays settled.

Then we introduce a bit of order to the cabin chaos. Louis inflates the dinghy and we tootle across to where the port policeman is waiting in his Land-rover. As I climb the ladder onto the quay I recognise the wild swaying sensation which is severe land-rock. I have to grip the Land Rover firmly while filling in the policeman's form, but he seems used to drunken sailors.

'Is there another round of formalities?' I ask, thinking of VAT. The official tells me there is a 'girl' who does the customs stuff but she's not here and she'll find us when she's ready. I'm hoping that if we plead that we're only here to land sick crew, they'll forgive us the lack of VAT.

The friendly official tells us that Paula's Place is the source of everything. We stagger up the near vertical hill, or so it seems, having seen nothing but flat for weeks, and find a little bar with some tables outside with people just finishing lunch. We find out immediately what our informant meant. Paula takes us under her wing. She finds some late lunch. Yes, washing can be taken in. Yes, diesel can be had in cans. Yes, water can be had. Yes, there is a cash machine up in the village. Yes, she will help me find Louis a flight home, a flight to Horta and then one onward. Yes, yes and yes, all very quietly, just how the traveller needs it. It transpires that Paula and her husband came to Flores from Connecticut, so we have something in common, though she and her husband are both Portuguese, he from the Azores originally, and she from Namibia.

On the way, there is an abandoned whaling skiff, the sort rowed by twelve men with Queequeg standing in the bows, harpoon poised, and Captain Ahab bellowing from the stern. It's perhaps thirty-five feet long and not more than six on the beam. It isn't seaworthy now but must have been in use within the last ten years. I remember that indigenous whalers are still allowed to hunt by hand. It goes against the grain but I have to admit that if they can deal with a full sized sperm whale from that filigree vessel, it seems fair game. There can't be many more bravely won dinners. Later, in one of the cafés, we see old black and white pictures of local whaling.

I suppose we must look a scruffy, dejected and rather pathetic crew when we wander into the courtyard because kind Paula observes our state of angst and sees to all our needs. What a find. She promises she will sort out diesel and water for us and assures us she can arrange for a woman in the village to do our washing, even when I explain that there are two enormous black bin bags full of damp, mildewed bedding and clothing, everything other than what we have on our backs. No problem. No problem.

Having listened to our worries and requests, Paula goes back in and returns with a tray of ice-cold, carbonated water in three misted pale green bottles. The snap and fizz of ice cold liquid on my tongue after weeks of tepid water is the best taste in the world, and I don't know whether to savour the sensation by rolling it round my mouth, or to down it so quickly that I numb my mouth and gullet. Because we have no idea that it is 4.30 p.m. local time, neither lunch nor supper, we ask for 'fish of the day' which is cooked and brought to us without complaint. Paula watches from her table as we guzzle down the cold liquid with sighs of pleasure, and tear fish off the bones. She is a canny woman. She seems to understand that we feel bewildered and very strange back on land after our voyage. She can sense my anxiety about my son and is not dismissive of it.

Louis is thin, drawn, and deathly pale even under the tan and beard. I know that he is in pain – in his bones and muscles and stomach. I see that he is too exhausted to speak and leave him to eat in silence. He looks like someone who is hanging on by a thread to hour-by-hour existence and he has to stay hanging or he will not manage to get home. His body aches for silence, solitude, darkness and the shutting down of all input but still he must keep going.

After the meal, we struggle on uphill until we come to a sprawling development of new houses, squat and boring with little patches of garden, a modern council estate with an ocean view. There we eventually find a bank and a supermarket with more empty shelves than stocked ones, and an empty cold store. No bread, eggs, meat, or fish. Unable to walk further, I sit on the pavement and wait while the other two walk to a second supermarket rumoured to be a further twenty minutes up the hill. I am sitting on the steps beneath the cash machine when the valiant Paula turns up in her car.

The other two arrive back with random things to eat, and Paula gives us all a lift back down to the harbour. I feel a strong connection with this woman and I think she feels the same way. We are both mothers.

Provisions in Lajes are sparse. We're mostly interested in fruit and vegetables but everyone gardens in the rich volcanic soil and warm damp climate, so there's no fresh produce in the shops. A sensible regime. We clear out what there is from both stores. The little local plums are intensely fruity, somewhere between a plum and a sweet damson. Absolutely delicious. We buy some fish and juice.

Louis and I swim from the boat in the harbour in sea skimmed with a rainbow of oil which shimmers in the sun.

After dinner, Stef takes the enormously heavy bags of wet washing up the hill to Paula's Place. I watch him from the boat, one black hefty bag balanced on his shoulders, one in his arms.

Louis goes ashore in the dinghy. I am reminded of E.T. phoning home. He stays in the phone box for a very, very long time.

CHAPTER 45

⚓

Travellers

The handful of cruising boats in the harbour is an interesting assembly of real travellers. There's an old Evasion with a high poop deck with a park bench across it and an inflatable crocodile in davits. This boat, we learn later, belongs to Manuel. We are about to set off for the shore the next day when we see him frantically waving as if drowning. He explains in Spanish something about losing his dinghy in a storm on the way from Bermuda and the croc is a replacement, and yes, he would prefer a lift in our boat if we're going his way. In addition to Manuel, there is a Dutchman with his Brazilian wife in a galleon type ketch; a sleek Kaufman 46 with an English couple aboard with whom we swap notes and get some useful tips about living with American boats in European electric zones; a French family with a sort of fish trap slung off the back of their sloop which holds the day's catch whilst the relevant references for cooking are looked up in Larousse; there's a sleek sloop with a highly experienced English couple aboard whom we later get talking to about refrigeration and the sailing life; and finally a Rival 34, not long in from Newport, with a young American family aboard. They left Newport a week or so before us, correctly synchronised with the depression, and even though their boat is ten feet shorter, they made the journey in not much over two weeks instead of our three. There's a lesson somewhere there. Next day the fleet is completed by an elegant 1950s teak 32 footer, with a couple of humorous German blokes aboard who seem to have trouble keeping clothes on. It appears to have about 2' 4" headroom so maybe it's not possible to get dressed.

Back aboard it's time for stocktaking. How did we do; a crew of beginners with a totally new boat on our first ocean outing? Setting aside Louis's illness, I'm quite pleased. We goofed our attempt to jump onto the weather roundabout on the east coast, and it, and the lack of a shakedown cruise, cost us a wet boat and a week of rolling around. But apart from the norther turning nor'easter, the weather could hardly have been kinder. Fifteen hundred miles close reaching with wind between 15 and 30 knots is a very fair hand to be dealt.

Our rations were adequate even losing the fridge. We would not have starved if the weather had been less ideal because we had lots of tins and dry stuff, although we would not have been ecstatic on that diet. This is a bit feeble against the history of maritime deprivations but we're a spoilt lot nowadays. As it turns out, the second and last tank of water runs out in Lajes harbour the day after we arrive, so we would have been down to the plastic jars of drinking water – about thirty gallons. We could have hung on for a while if we'd been becalmed. I thought we had been very conservative with water so I'm a bit chastened that the three of us have all but dried the tanks out.

As far as gear is concerned, the broken alternator bracket is by far the most serious problem. There appear to be virtually no facilities in Lajes. We could probably get a car mechanic to have a look. It's a welding job, and not an easy one, stainless to rustable. Worse, it would be hard to reach the part to be welded from a welding rig on the jetty. All the boats have to be kept a few feet away from the jetty because of the big ocean swells. They're a resourceful lot here, but it might take time getting it all together. The jury rig lash-up we put together appears to be working well and the batteries are fully charged. We've only used about fifteen gallons of diesel the whole trip – a little under 200 miles per US gallon – which we now replenish from jars brought down from the local filling station. I really don't want to go to Horta for repairs and wind up paying more than £10K VAT for the privilege of a three day stopover, so it looks as if the alternator jury rig will be tested on the Canaries leg too. Louis's fix of the mast-track seems fine.

Will the insurance cover us without Louis? A fine point! I don't think a reasonable company would blame us since we fully expected to have three aboard and have dropped him off because of illness. I suppose they might argue that we should have taken on replacement crew in the Azores. That wouldn't be easy, certainly not in Lajes. The crew shortage is mainly an issue for watch keeping, and since we will only be crossing one shipping lane all the way from here to the Canaries, with a journey of one week rather than three, it seems reasonable to proceed.

Sunday 10th July

After a whole night of sound sleep in a bed which neither rocks nor tips me on to the floor, I wake restored and leap on deck to take in my surroundings. Yesterday was a blur. People are up and about, the two Germans sitting in their cockpit, naked, shaving and washing and drinking coffee; Manuel is tidying his boat; others are hanging out washing or pottering about on deck. Boat people, like us.

Louis needs space and silence to pack so Stef and I set off in search of supplies forgetting that it is Sunday and everywhere is shut.

Schlepping uphill, just in case the second supermarket is open, we are set upon by several crazy Rottweiler that leap into the lane barking and snarling, creeping up on us and backing off. I cling to Stef's arm. On the way back from the supermarket – closed, of course – I insist we cross a lumpy field to avoid the dogs but our diversion ends in a wall too high to scale so we retrace our steps and meet the vicious dogs again. Ignore them, Stef says, walking on briskly as if they were not there.

Back down the steep hill, near to Paula's Place, we find that the little bar that was closed on the way up is open now. While Stef hovers impatiently outside, I go in and ask for ice. After much sign language and intervention from a man who speaks a little English, my request is understood; the barman empties his ice-machine into polythene bags for me. Then I spot the cakes – chocolate eclairs and apple pie. Yes, please. Off we go again, with ridiculously thin poly bags of rapidly melting ice hanging from our fingers, and goodies for tea.

Back at the boat, Louis sits beside his enormous rucksack, ready to leave even though his plane is not until tomorrow. I sense that he has already left us and has cut loose so that he can make the transition and cope with the tough journey ahead. I watch him trying to conserve every ounce of energy because he is running on empty. He is desperate to get off the boat – for his own survival and because he is distraught that his health has not held up. This was to be a significant trial and a test of his journey towards recovery, and we all know that it has failed. I sense that he feels personal failure, as if it were somehow his fault. I want to tell him that the illness is to blame. The energy levels required for this kind of challenge were not there. The mood on the boat is sombre and sad. We are all waiting for the moment when Louis leaves.

In the evening the three of us climb down into the dinghy to go ashore for the last time. Stef and I feel wretched for our son, but even as we hide our feelings, we know that he knows exactly how we feel. We climb the hill to Paula's where folk from the other boats have already gathered at the tables outside, drinking beer, eating, shouting and laughing. Paula, tuned in to our son's distress, brings him a huge platter of steak, eggs and chips while Stef and I eat baked fish. It is a good last meal together. We toast the end of our voyage, toast Scarlet, and wish Louis all the luck in the world in getting home safely. We collect our dry, folded laundry and Paula books a taxi for early the following morning.

As we are leaving, Paula says, 'I really like you guys, you know.'

She seems oddly attached to us. Maybe it is the wretchedness which leaks through our social masks and the sadness that hangs about us. She takes Louis's face in her hands and compares it to Stef's.

'You can tell who is his daddy! The same mouth, eyes. Not the same nose. His . . .' pointing at Stef's nose, '. . . is sharper.'

'For getting stones out of horses' hooves,' he replies, his stock response, but completely lost in translation.

We discuss features for a bit and she teases me that none of my genes have reached my son, and I disagree silently, knowing that the genes that trigger ME have passed from me to him. However, such thoughts are way beyond pidgin Portuguese and sign language, so I just sigh to myself.

Tomorrow I will regret not having thanked Paula properly for her motherly kindness. I do not know that I won't see her again. I do not know that when Louis has left, Stef and I will feel an urgent need to leave too. We are running away from the pain.

CHAPTER 46

Louis leaves Scarlet

MONDAY 11TH JULY

I surface at 8.45 a.m., ready to wake Louis, there he is, pale and wan, face like a white mask, sitting on deck with his rucksack.

'You're up early,' I say stupidly.

'Never went to sleep,' he replies.

'Oh no. Why?'

'Just too ill.'

This damn ME. The more tired you get, the more impossible it is to sleep or unwind. The body is stuck in the fright and flight state with adrenalin pulsing round the body making rest and relaxation impossible. A perpetual fairground ride without any of the fun. The 'fatigue' of 'chronic fatigue', its popular name in the UK, could not be more of a misnomer.

Stef and Louis climb down to the dinghy and Louis pulls the cord to start the motor. I wave to them as they chug to the shore, then notice that Louis has left his sandals behind. Will he walk barefoot back to the UK? He has a horrible journey ahead because the only route we could find at the last minute involves three planes and an overnight wait in an airport. My heart is heavy with worry for him, my sick son. We should not have taken him with us on this crossing. This has become my constant refrain.

When Stef returns, heavy hearted and sad, he tells me that the taxi was already waiting and that Louis is now on his way. Good for Paula; she arranged everything just as she promised, including lending Stef the clapped out Volvo van so that he could fetch diesel from the petrol station owned by her husband. Back at the jetty, Stef unloads fifteen large, assorted plastic cans of diesel into the dinghy.

I row Louis ashore for his taxi to the airport and see him on his way with a heavy heart. I hate to lose him, especially in the circumstance of him becoming ill again. We would not have got here without him and while he thrived for the first half of the trip, his heroic efforts to sort the genoa while repeatedly soaked in cold water has brought on a relapse. It's my fault. And he has a long and arduous journey ahead with an overnight wait on Horta. Not the best road to recovery.

I am on the boat washing clothes – a chore to occupy my hands while my mind is troubled and unsettled – when I see two dinghies approaching. Stef is being towed by our friends from Express Crusader, the yacht deliverers, now delivering Stef and cans of diesel because he ran out of dinghy fuel in the middle of the bay.

'Shameful!' I shout as they come alongside.

They lend us their funnel so that Stef can pour the diesel into our tanks, and because he has bought too much, he can at least give them what is left in thanks. They take the extra full tanks, and all the empty ones, and zip off again. They are having such fun, those two, although the previous night at Paula's, they told us that they were giving up this crazy way of living and are planning to buy a farm instead. They have been on the seas for about twenty years delivering yachts to all parts of the world.

Next – water. Paula has arranged this too. We have never had water delivered to the boat by a fire engine, but that's how it is done on Flores, in return for a contribution to the local brigade. We prepare to move Scarlet to the dock to wait. The fire engine is due some time in the afternoon and arrives, as promised, about 4 p.m. Lots and lots of water!

*

I am at the helm, ready for the last leg, and steer Scarlet gently away from the pier. I am proud of my manoeuvre, but as I smugly move out into the bay, weaving between the other yachts, I see that I have left my husband standing on the dock with a rope in his hands making big gestures of exasperation. Oops! Scarlet has to be turned round and squeezed back against the dock so that he can jump aboard, but it is not easy because the length of the dock is not much bigger than our own length, and a good six feet above our deck.

As men feel free to do when there is a woman at the wheel, Stef screams instructions at me from the dock.

'To port!'

'To starboard!'

'Slow down! SLOW DOWN!'

'Starboard!'

'SLOWER!'

Other men join him until there is a whole line of them, all shouting at me in different languages. It is impossible to make out a single word. Only those of my husband.

'For fuck's sake, slow down!'

'Oh do shut up!' I yell back, in a snap of bad temper. 'Or I'll leave you there and go on alone!'

Finally I am close enough for him to jump down from the dock and, with an almighty bang wallop, he lands on the deck.

I block my ears to his foul language.

CHAPTER 47

Crew of Two

Just the two of us now!

Lurking around the harbour wall is a frigate of the Portuguese line. Isn't that a bit excessive for collecting unpaid VAT from a yacht? The sailors are all lined up on the afterdeck, looking for all the world as if they're having a lecture on fishing from an officer with a rod in his hand. Fly casting on the afterdeck? Perhaps it's a whip antenna to illustrate a signals lecture? Anyway, whatever it is, it's sufficiently distracting that they forget about our VAT.

A week later, back home we will hear that Louis saw us heading out of Lajes harbour, looking down from his flight out to Horta.

We hoist the sails, set course for the north with a wind west of north. It's a great sail. As evening arrives, we slowly start to unwind, letting go of the tension and angst that has filled the past days. How can it be otherwise, sailing off again on the next leg of our journey, the wind and the ocean behaving themselves and helping us on our way?

We set off from Flores in bright sun and a fine light breeze which gives us an idyllic reach. *Ocean Passages* tells us that the main hazard of this leg of the journey is cutting corners and winding up becalmed too near the centre of the Azores high, especially at the beginning when trying to get away from the islands. The first one hundred and fifty miles will see us pass north of Graciosa, San Jorge and Terceira in a long arc, and then the same again to pass San Miguel and exit from the archipelago, passing Madeira en route to the Canaries.

It's the best part of a thousand miles to Tenerife, keeping Madeira about a hundred miles to port towards the end of the trip. We nonchalantly treat this as a day trip. We are heading for Tenerife mainly because we know there are good direct flights home. In retrospect it would have been wiser to head up for the windward Lanzarote, to leave our round-Canaries options open. We didn't do our homework on the Canaries before leaving nearly as thoroughly as we should because it seemed presumptuous to plan the journey in greater detail. Why? I notice this is a refrain in my nautical planning. Inasmuch as we have long term plans, they are to spend perhaps a year's holidays exploring the Canaries and getting to know· the boat and then head for the Caribbean.

This is easy sailing. We both relax. The boat and all our bedding are fresh and bone dry. Batteries and tanks are full and cupboards full enough. Scarlet seems to know exactly what to do. We're sailing effortlessly, between 6 and 7 knots on a broad reach. The frigate passes us a couple of miles to the South, steaming at perhaps 20 knots, fishing lesson finished. We feel not a hint of trepidation. What's a thousand miles for a couple of old salts? We're two-thousand-miles-a-leg sailors now!

Tuesday 12th July

The clouds roll in but we are sailing on in a quiet, relaxed way. Stef and I have slotted back into our familiar roles of captain and first mate, and, without Louis, I have taken back the chores and responsibilities which he had taken from me. We meet no challenges so the extra responsibility is fine.

Relieved of the hour by hour monitoring of the declining health of my son and the guilt that accompanied it, I breathe out. I'm still worrying about him – I always do – but the anxiety is at one remove. My son is very ill and there is nothing I can do.

The start of this leg of the journey is calm and wonderfully uneventful. Almost boring – but Stefan and I don't do bored. Day follows day. The sun rises, crosses the sky and sets. Stefan and I interact as we have always done when we are a crew of two. We move around one another with quiet ease, coming together for meals, or to sit on deck and talk. The past crossing is too recent to have gelled into distinct memories or distinct emotions. Later, we will go over and over it. For now, in the evenings, we read Simenon's Maigret in French, out loud, lying stretched out on the captain's bunk. Partly it's to while away the time. Partly we have become addicted to the Maigret crime stories.

That first evening, we set course to round the next island. As night closes in, I sit on deck watching the lights on land. We pass one lighthouse. Then another. Scarlet is sailing beautifully and by midnight the island is a blur of fairy lights far behind us.

Eventually, we find we cannot sustain our easterly course between the islands. We need to turn back and go round the back of them. Stef has trouble on night watch with ships turning into lighthouses and lighthouses turning into ships.

Friday 15th July

We have slowed right down. Stef and I spend all day trying different sail settings and combinations, including the genoa on the spinnaker pole but to no avail.

We decide to take the genoa off the pole because it is behaving no better than it does flying out with sheets. In one split second the big sail blows right out of our hands, out of our reach, and twists itself round and round and round the forstay, not in any coherent, rolled up fashion, but this way then that way until it is so tightly wrapped it is impossible to prise it free.

Stef battles with the sail for almost an hour, but each time he gets a piece of it free, and is hanging on to a corner of the stiff fabric for dear life, the wind whips it out of his hands and wraps it round the forstay again. Talk about knickers in a twist. Then the sail lashes out and winds itself round Stef's arm and starts a tug of war, dragging him in its grasp towards the side of the bows.

'My arm!' He shouts. 'My arm is trapped. I can't get it free.'

Oh my God! The sail is shaking itself to pieces and with it, Stef's arm. He will be lifted off the deck and wrapped round the forstay himself. Then he will be spat out into the ocean, with or without his arm still attached to his body. These things happen. I have seen quite a few sailors minus an arm or hand. But in a lull, Stef manages to extract his arm. Shocked and winded, he sits on deck and rests while I watch the damn genoa flap itself into a rhythm of coil-uncoil, coil-uncoil, never ending.

Watching these maddening repetitions, I finally see that there is a not just a rhythmic motion but a clear pattern to the sail's frantic winding and unwinding. Each time the wind catches it, it winds clockwise, then, as the wind drops, anti-clockwise again. I realise that it is pointless fighting it when the wind has it in its power. I tell Stef that he needs to unwind only in the moments when it is not spinning. We both go back to the bows and this time he battles with the sail only when I shout, 'Now! And now!' It works, the sail is loose, but it is a close call because we could have had the genoa twisted so tightly that it would never have come loose.

Back in the cockpit, we register how much our backs and arms ache, and how winded we are. I cook chorizo with fried red peppers out of a jar, tinned tomatoes and rice.

We don't bother keeping watch. We lie down and are instantly asleep.

Saturday 16th July
There is very little wind. I bribe Stef to put the motor on for a couple of hours.

'Come on,' I say. 'Let's block our ears under the sheet for a while.'

Afterwards, because the engine has been running, I have the self-indulgent, sensual luxury of washing my hair in hot water and soaping my sticky skin. Later, we eat rice with very old chorizo and tinned okra.

With no spare fan belts left, Stef has been painstakingly splicing a rope which might work as a substitute. Now he fits it and tells me to stand back while he fires up the engine. The rope lasts twenty seconds before it is ripped to shreds. Dire warnings from Stef now: the engine only just started; if we try to start the engine again, it may fire or it may not. We don't know if there is any power left in the battery. I feel contrite after persuading him to run the motor because he would not have done it otherwise. With current conditions it will take us four or five more days to reach the Canaries and our food cupboard is almost bare. And I've just finished my very last novel I have on board.

Night falls. No instruments. No GPS. No lights.

Sunday July 17th

I wake late to a square of blue sky in the shape of my overhead hatch, and hear water sloshing peacefully past the boat. Once so vigilant, Stef and I have become careless about night watches but sleep is beautiful. I open the hatch a squeak – no more salt water in my bed please – and see that the sea is the right shade of blue with enough crisscross lines and toothpaste foam to indicate the right amount of wind.

I fry tinned ham and home-made bread in olive oil for Stef who declares it the best fried bread he has ever eaten.

⚓

CHAPTER 48

Dead batteries

The steady breeze continues for the rest of the night. Just before dawn we can see the light on São Jorge and soon, in the dawn, the unlit Graciosa.

Later in the day, when Terceira comes into view, the wind picks up to 15 knots and by nightfall it's 20 and then 25. The nightfall factor is always worth a few extra knots in the psychological reckoning of wind speed but even allowing for this, finding enough wind to get off the archipelago doesn't seem to be our problem. I begin to consider cutting south of San Miguel. We can make north of San Miguel on a close reach, but it's a lee shore with some substantial Atlantic breakers bearing down, and lee shores give me the shudders. On the other hand, south of San Miguel, in the gap between Terceira and San Miguel, there's D. João de Castro Bank which, at twelve metres deep, hardly counts as water, and further on there's the unlit Ilheus das Formigas. Perhaps with the big seas coming down from the NE it will get ugly over those shallows?

I'm thinking conservatively – both routes would probably be fine – but this is the first choice of route I have made in 1500 miles so I make a meal of it. It's part of getting back into coastal sailing mode. We opt for the southerly route just before I hand over to Lynn. As it turns out, the wind drops and backs 15 degrees during her watch, so she decides to revert to the northerly route. We don't see anything of San Miguel except the powerful beam of the lighthouse as we depart the eastern tip.

I'm back on watch and spend a night staring at bewildering illuminations.

There seems to be a lighthouse about fifty miles north of San Miguel. It isn't on the chart, nor anything for it to stand on, and it's far too deep there to drill for anything except sea water with which the good Burghers of San Miguel are already well supplied. It is probably a fishing boat producing the illusion of a light pattern rising and falling in the regular swell. A little later, there is a whole array of lights of varying hues engaged in formation dancing. I eventually put these down to pair of trawlers but not before going through the full range of shipping constellations like barges on the Mississippi and all that stuff from the Yachtmaster course. It's strange how the mind goes for definite options on such flaky evidence. A couple of lights and a few reflections off a superstructure and my brain has conjured up a whole fishing village on Ilheus das Formigas, even though it would have to be twenty miles off the usual pitch and our information tells us there are no villages, fishing or otherwise. Full blown hallucination would come effortlessly at sea.

By the end of my watch we're well past Santa Maria with its lighthouse – the last remnant of the Azores – and Scarlet is on a broad reach with the bit between her willful teeth. She feels just like the racehorses I occasionally helped exercise many years ago. They only had one idea and that was GO! The trick was to try to keep them in their early morning dozy and befuddled state while walking to the beach. They were telepathic so it was crucial that you didn't even think of anything the least bit exciting until you hit the sands. Then they would explode from asleep to full speed in three strides. In similar vein, we have cajoled Scarlet with a gentle touch until she passes the last rocks off the Azores and then, smelling the full breadth of the Atlantic, she's off. Don't try pulling on her reins now! Unless you want to loosen your arms in their sockets.

She knocks off two 170 mile days, barely consulting us. The Minotaur is her accomplice which demands not so much as a tweak of its string. On the third day Scarlet pauses for breath while the wind moderates, and then she's off for another couple of 170s.

I can't bear to run the engine to charge the batteries because it will disturb the peace. We're being careful with juice but even so the batteries are down to about half full. I eventually fire it up and check the diodes to see that the alternator is charging. An hour later I check again to see how many amp-hours have gone in to find that the alternator has stopped charging. Oh, that sinking feeling! Inspection shows that the alternator belt has gone again. Too much vibration for the last and final belt.

This is not good, though not immediately life-threatening. We are perhaps three days away from Tenerife and we needn't run anything other than navigation lights during the short July nights. We don't need any of the wind instruments or the autopilot. Bless the Minotaur again! We have the Gecko for position, and the chart plotter doesn't take much juice for an occasional double check. The depth sounder might be useful for getting into a marina, and maybe a bit of VHF at the end. The engine starting battery is separate and should be charged, so we shouldn't need to engage in the heroics of sailing into the marina.

The last two days are more of the same, blissful progress with all credit to boat and wind vane and little to the crew. We pass Madeira well out of sight off the port beam and I think how pleasant it would be to make a leisurely visit. But delivery skippers cannot mooch about. Finally we pick up the loom of the lighthouse on the north western tip of Tenerife.

It's the evening of the eighth day out from Flores.

CHAPTER 49

Movers and shakers

By the time I come on watch at midnight the wind has picked up to 20 knots. We were always expecting an interesting passage around this corner of the island where Teide, the extinct volcano which is Tenerife, rises 2400 metres out of the water, accelerating the prevailing NE wind and bending it to the north or even the northwest. With the wind at 20 knots out here, I predict that we will be hit by a full gale as we round the corner, and sure enough the build up soon begins. Teide has plans for the crescendo of our voyage.

We reduce the mainsail to the third reef, and roll up all but a third of the genoa. Despite giving the lighthouse a good seven mile berth we have started to surf across the steepening swell.

At this corner of the island the Canary current, built up in the fetch of a thousand miles of north easterlies, is climbing the slope and ridging its back with the effort. Although there is more than 800 meters of water in the channel, there is 4500 meters of water where we have just come from. I time the knot meter at 10 knots for a sustained period of more than a minute. Our hull speed, the speed the hull can be driven through the water without climbing out, is less than nine.

The wind reaches 37 knots. During this surge, Scarlet is vibrating like a wild animal straining its muscles, and making an alarming noise midway between humming and roaring: a wild mare indeed. I am hoping that we don't have to bring her round to lose speed, but much more of this and that is what it will have to be. We have seven miles of sea between us and the point, but the worry is broaching – getting pushed around sideways on to the wind as we surf down the back of each towering roller.

Scarlet is shuddering and trembling as if she is about to burst every seam in her body before scattering herself across the sea. Then, just as we reach a crazy pitch and I start thinking about what is going to happen when I disengage the Minotaur, the wind passes its crescendo. Over the next half mile, it drops to nothing. And I mean nothing. Flat calm. We ghost along with the sails flapping, slower and slower, until we come to a dead, rolling halt. There is a considerable sea running but not a breath of wind. We're under the volcano. That innocent looking corner of the island provided a truly Shakespearean climax. The strongest wind, the nastiest sea and the highest speed we have experienced during the entire trip across the ocean.

Pathos followed by bathos. We're rolling about, only thirty miles from Los Cristianos which is our destination and, not in the mood for being churned to butter, I reach to switch on the engine.

Wah! Wah! Wahuuuurgh.

The starting battery is flat. I switch the almost flat house batteries into the engine starter motor circuit to give that little extra push.

One more Wah!' but barely a Wahuuuurgh.

We have no engine. Now what? Why is our engine-starting battery not as separate as it is supposed to be? That question will have to wait.

We spend several horrible, uncomfortable hours trying to find some wind. We succeed, but only by being washed back into the maelstrom that just spat us out. Again it shakes us until our teeth are loose and spits us out into the identical place after another spell of trembling and shuddering. We could be at this for a while. I fancy that the volcano's wind shadow is stationary as long as the wind stays in the NE, which is all the summer months and most of the winter too. No doubt local knowledge knows just how far over to Gomera we should have held our course to sail around this black vortex, but I can't find any information in the pilot. We could wallow and shake indefinitely, but it is getting late and we are feeling done in.

I can take no more. I swear Scarlet will shake herself to pieces and we will be blown on to the rocks as flotsam. Ignoring Stefan's incredible hesitation,

I get on the VHF. I use the last gasp of the battery to ask to be rescued. We wallow for a couple more hours and then a vessel appears as a bright orange spot a long way off but heading our way. Oh, the shame! Men in fluorescent safety gear clamber aboard. The salvage vessel from Los Cristianos hitches us up and tows Scarlet for three ignominious hours the entire length of the southern coast of Tenerife. Stefan is silent. Me too. We stare at the horizon pretending that this isn't really happening. Stefan looks like he wishes the ocean would swallow him. 'Sorry, Scarlet,' I whisper. It was never meant to end like this. We were supposed to motor triumphantly into the harbour after clocking up 3000 miles and surviving to tell the tale. It will take a few days to recover from this pathetic anticlimax and to hammer the dents out of our pride.

In front of the usual mocking, gawping audience that gathers for these events, we are being helped to tie Scarlet to the jetty behind the high sea wall. They probably think we are amateurs on holiday. All the other yachts are at anchor in the bay so everyone can see that ours is the boat that had to be rescued. Oh the shame.

Lynn goes around in a hat and sunglasses, pretending that this boat – the only one tied up to the jetty wall – is not hers. Each time she returns from foraging, I watch her wait until the coast is clear before doing a runner towards Scarlet. As a punishment, I take the jokes and banter from sailors and bystanders on the chin.

I don't explain that we have just crossed an ocean.

Epilogue

⚓

2011

We would have written this account even if we always knew it was destined for the filing cabinet. I write mainly to find out what I think and feel about things. People who aren't in the habit of writing – even if only letters or emails or diaries or memos – find this odd. They would argue that once you know what you think or feel, then you write it down. But this isn't how I, and other writers I know, experience it. It's the writing that helps shape the thought, at least on good days, and on bad days when words can't be found or put in an order, the causality goes the other way. On those days I know that the reason I can't write is that the thought is not yet thought.

Looking back, one of the greatest satisfactions was being part of a family pack that pulled together and worked quietly to make conditions tolerable. Apart from the sticky patch when we could not agree whether we were continuing to the Azores, turning back to Long Island or heading for Bermuda, there was hardly a cross word. For Lynn and me, the most harrowing outcome is knowing that this journey has made Louis very ill. I only hope he will come back to life with rest. Two steps forward, one to three steps back – an all too familiar dance. I sense how much he has grown up. He is much older now than when he arrived in the boatyard. Our son has been superb all the way through.

Lynn has stuck it out 'downstairs' in the churning washing drum, serving up food. I'm useless downstairs at sea. I can navigate when I have to, but otherwise my two modes at sea are either on deck or asleep (or asleep on deck). There are no extra functions on this model. But cooking was the least of Lynn's contributions. Remaining cheerful, even excited, was a more difficult trick, and she never failed. Bizarrely, she had faith in the captain and his navigator, something unnerving rather than reassuring. If she only knew what I know, she'd be throwing the switch on the EPIRB, I thought several times in bleaker moments. But her trust was a huge contribution.

In the family pack, each of us sensed what needed doing and did it. The best feeling in the world. Of course, there was the occasional, usually hilarious, misunderstanding, or 'mutual delegation,' but rare, and never any recrimination. The feeling of oneness is much magnified at sea because of the total immersion – in the journey, not the water, though that too at times. At home, where our immediate safety is not an issue, being in tune with the needs and feelings of others is not so common nor so intense. While responsible for the others and the boat, I was perhaps not very good at emerging from this total immersion to voice my positive reflections and to give the other two the acknowledgement they deserved. I can here.

One regret is that this book is lopsidedly written by the older generation. Louis's voyage was different again, and it leaves a story untold, but he has better things to do than to go in search of time past, and he doesn't share his parents' obsession with scribbling. I think he has added one sentence somewhere in the middle. Did you find it?

We have sold Scarlet.

After reaching the Canaries, we came home and settled down to land-life for a while. But then we were informed that Scarlet was taking up a parking space reserved for yachts competing in the ARC 2006. We were given two choices: fly out from Scotland and move her within the next month or pay our dues and be added to the list of boats who would race across the Atlantic to St Lucia. We didn't want to cross that stretch of ocean again because the first time had been so memorable, but because of work commitments we couldn't manage the first option so reluctantly, we became part of the jamboree. We wanted to get to the Caribbean so we decided to do it this way. And a bit of a shock it was. Yachts ranged from sleek, brand new 80 footers with uniformed crew who polished the brightwork from morning til night to us in our grotty shorts and a few eccentrics who took part because they liked running the Pub Quiz each evening. There was singing and dancing and speeches, and when the starting gun went off, two hundred and fifty boats milled around the starting line. That was pretty much the last we saw of them. It was a tedious trip with the wind behind us and Scarlet rocking right, rocking left, rocking right. Arriving was good though. As we sailed into Rodney Bay, the crews on the yachts that has beaten us (most) rang their bells and hooted and yelled.

For a year or so, we continued to fly out to the Caribbean in the holidays and sailed around the beautiful islands. We swam in turquoise waters. But the harsh Caribbean sun and gales and torrential rains were taking their toll on Scarlet. The damage mounted. So we hauled her out in a boatyard in Trinidad and flew out for another two years but spent all our time scraping and re-varnishing wood and getting the rust off the brightwork with brillo pads. It was a full time job. We lived and worked in the boatyard. We didn't sail.

In the end, we could not justify keeping her. The costs of the boatyard and the costs of replacement parts were prohibitive, as were the long haul flights twice a year. We didn't like the impact on the planet of flying such distances. Our plan had been to hang on to Scarlet until we could carry out our cherished plan of living aboard and sailing round the world, but one very elderly father had not departed for the next land so we couldn't go anywhere either. Now in our sixties, and the Aged P still with us, it is too late for that adventure.

We sold Scarlet.

Then we sold our Edinburgh flat and set off for southern France to build a self-sustaining house there. It was Plan B and even that didn't quite happen. We fell in love with a half-built house with breathtaking views across vineyards and towards mountains. We have exterior walls and a habitable top floor. The downstairs is the biggest garage in Langedoc, full of dirt and rubble and a cement mixer. We are living on a building site in the sun.

Stef made himself at home in two minutes. He has not looked back. After thirty-two years in the same Edinburgh academic department, he walked away from his day job and never looked back. I have been slower.

I ricochet between Scotland and France, reluctant to drag my young publishing house away from the literary city, equally reluctant to leave my colleagues and friends. But the blus skies and my wish to leave behind the frantic pace and madness of life in the UK is winning me round.

Stef has bought himself a second-hand digger. He is building a swimming pool on a perilous slope which he is propping up with about thirty massive rock-filled gabions. He is back to his old tricks – impossible projects that require very hard physical toil. Inside, perched on a stool, he has drilled away the downstairs ceiling – all 130 square metres of it – and is running miles of rigid piping up and down, up and down, to create low energy under-floor heating. And it's only cold for two months! I am trying to create a home in the light-filled, open-plan space upstairs and am making a garden out of rock and boulders and builders' rubble. We live in a clearing in an oak forest, and nothing puts down roots here. Will we?

While we labour, we won't forget our other adventure. I wrote this log as we were approaching Tenerife. It is my last tribute to the blue boat called Scarlet that carried us safely across the ocean.

*

There is almost no food left, and no electricity therefore no instruments because we dare not turn on the engine. Stef reckons there is enough charge in the battery for one last attempt to start it, maybe two, in an emergency. The gib is nothing more than long raggedy strips that flutter like ribbons on a Maypole. But who cares? For now, the mainsail is set just so and we are moving with grace through the just-right-blue sea.

I go and sit as far forward as I can in the bows. This has been a forbidden place for much of the trip – too wet, too bumpy, too dangerous. I have only just settled when I see a shoal of dolphins alongside the boat. They are so close I can imagine stretching out a hand to stroke their glistening, spotted skins. They dip and dive, jump in arcs and even shoot straight out of the water until their curiosity is satisfied and, at a sign from one of them perhaps, in formation they swim away.

I stand in the bows, wind in my hair, on my face and arms, toasted warm by the sun. Three years ago today my mother died. She loved the sea. She would have loved being on this boat. I try to find a word for today: simple, blue, perfect.

No, the best word for today is Scarlet.

This book is a message in a bottle. When we wrote it, it was not clear whether it would ever find an audience or just sink into the abyss over which we had just sailed so memorably. There was no guarantee that the message would reach others nor that they would read it and respond. Messages in bottles suggest we are happy to leave things to chance and serendipity.